CAN YOU DIE OF A BROKEN HEART?

CAN YOU DIE OF A BROKEN HEART?

A heart surgeon's insight into what makes us tick

DR NIKKI STAMP

MURDOCH BOOKS

SYDNEY · LONDON

Published in 2018 by Murdoch Books,
an imprint of Allen & Unwin

Murdoch Books Australia
83 Alexander Street, Crows Nest NSW 2065
Phone: +61 (0)2 8425 0100
murdochbooks.com.au
info@murdochbooks.com.au

Murdoch Books UK
Ormond House, 26–27 Boswell Street, London WC1N 3JZ
Phone: +44 (0) 20 8785 5995
murdochbooks.co.uk
info@murdochbooks.co.uk

For corporate orders and custom publishing contact our business
development team at salesenquiries@murdochbooks.com.au

Copyright © Nikki Stamp 2018
Publisher: Jane Morrow
Editorial Manager: Jane Price
Design Manager: Madeleine Kane
Editor: Meaghan Amor
Author photography: Chris Chen

ISBN 978 1 76063 166 6 Australia
ISBN 978 1 76063 425 4 UK

A cataloguing-in-publication entry is available from the catalogue
of the National Library of Australia at nla.gov.au
A catalogue record for this book is available from the British Library

Chapter opener illustration shows the Olson Acoustic Stethoscope 1943

Printed and bound in Glasgow by MBM Print SCS Ltd.

10 9 8 7 6 5 4 3 2 1

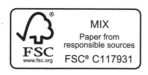

MIX
Paper from
responsible sources
FSC® C117931

For Taolo Masilonyane-Jones

A gentleman and a scholar
Missed always

CONTENTS

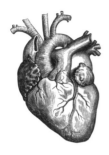

introduction:
WHAT IS IT ABOUT THE HEART?

When was the last time you thought about how your body works on the inside? Have you ever stopped to imagine how the air moves in and out of your chest? Maybe you've wondered how your brain tells your muscles to move so you can walk. Have you lain awake, aware of your heartbeat, and pondered how your heart knows when to be fast and when to be slow? It's not something we do very often, largely because we don't need to.

The thing about our bodies is that a lot goes on behind the scenes. You don't have to tell your heart to beat or your lungs to breathe. Your gut just processes the food you present and, when you want to walk, your brain simply has your legs get on with it. It's easy to take it all for granted. The thing is, our bodies are amazing and we don't stop often enough to appreciate just how fantastic they are.

Since I was a child I've been fascinated by the way the body works. As an adult and a heart surgeon, I've narrowed that obsession to just the chest. In folklore and ancient medicine the heart was always seen as a magical life-giving core and that is exactly how I feel about it. Now I want to share some of the magic and knowledge of that organ that thumps away in your chest, that you feel flutter when you're excited and pound when you're nervous. I want you to love your heart so much that you take care of it with your mind, body and soul. I feel fortunate to be able to look at hearts virtually every day of my life and I am on a mission to make sure you find the heart as fascinating and precious as I do. I want to take you on a journey to learn how your heart beats and how to make every one of those beats count.

The heart is, at its simplest, a pump. A pump, and also a kind of enigma: its simplicity is possible because of complexities that we're only just learning about. The heart is put together in such a way that it just works beautifully.

Heart surgery has only been in existence for about 60 years. Before that we didn't know enough about the heart to cut it open, fix it and then put it back together again. As recently as 1912, a doctor by the name of Stephen Paget remarked that we had reached the pinnacle of knowledge and skill relating to the heart. He considered the heart so vital, so life-sustaining, that we could not afford to be charging into the chest to understand and repair its inner workings – unlike the progress being made in other areas of medicine and surgery at the time. This assumption turned out to be wrong; what we can now do to fix broken hearts is incredible.

Since 400 BC anatomists and philosophers have debated the significance of the heart. Aristotle rightly deduced that it was the centre of the body's circulation and a vital organ. Over the centuries the brightest minds have sought to understand the heart – both its physical side and its spiritual.

I would like to introduce the heart and all the features that make it beautiful, special and healthy. I'll explain how being depressed can make it sick, but a good night's sleep can make it healthy. I'd also like to share the stories of some amazing heart-owners I've met in my work as a surgeon.

I don't intend to provide you with a list of things you must do to be healthy or a plan to follow, set out day by day. I want to share my fascination with you. My hope is that you will be as captivated by the workings of the heart as I am. I am wagering that if you know how amazing your own heart is, you will want to care for it every day.

Your heart is your own and it can do incredible things. It's beating inside your chest, pumping blood, feeling fear and helping you run. I want to explain some of what I know about this little ball of muscle and show you how to love this beautiful organ, physically and emotionally. Not a plan or a how-to guide, but rather a kind of show-and-tell – so you can fall in love with your heart and look after its every beautiful beat.

My path to the heart

As a child I was fascinated by the way the human body was put together and how all those cogs fitted to become this glorious machine. I simply could not devour enough information about the organs: how the heart beat, the lungs breathed, the eye saw the world around us and even how poo was made. Don't misunderstand me, I read just as much *Baby-Sitters Club* as the next little girl, but it was the books on our bodies that truly made me tick. I read anatomy books, books on the heart, the eye and the bones. I knew the first-aid manuals backwards and I was ready to jump into action at a moment's notice.

When I was six or seven my mother was contacted by the primary school librarian to express concern that I wasn't reading appropriate books for my age; by that we think she meant more Enid Blyton, less anatomy. Fast forward 20-something years and that fascination has never disappeared, but has become a career. Now, rather than poring over books and pictures, I see hearts most days of my life as a cardiothoracic surgeon – a surgeon who cares for the heart and the lungs. I feel incredibly fortunate to be able to fix broken hearts.

My path to the heart wasn't exactly straightforward. I desperately wanted a career in musical theatre, but my pragmatic engineer-father suggested (insisted) that I get a 'real' degree first. So, I was going to study accountancy; however, a brief illness and hospital admission just before my final high-school exams made me realise that balance sheets were not for me and there was something else I wanted to do. My experience as a patient, seeing hospital staff who were wrapped up in the world of the human body – its workings, its failings, along with the very human side of what it is to care for another person – inspired me to put accounting at the bottom of the list.

Solely focused on treading the boards and not believing in my academic aptitude, I thought many career options were out of the question for me. My dad took away the growing pile of university prospectuses and course outlines and asked me a very simple question: 'If you could do anything in the world, regardless of marks or subjects, what would it be?' To both our surprise, without a moment's hesitation, my response was medicine. Somewhere my brain had remembered that childhood fascination. I set about working to get into medicine at this late stage. It was no easy road, but I did it and I have never looked back.

Perhaps without realising, I was always going to be a surgeon. I could blame it squarely on growing up in a house with an engineering father who was always fixing or making things; he even built his own yacht. In our lounge room. Couple that with my mum's extraordinary attention to detail and her way with language and communications, and they created a surgeon. I loved the way surgery could make a real, immediate and measureable change to someone's life. A tumour, gone; a blockage, bypassed; pain, all banished with the scalpel and a deft pair of hands.

Heart surgery, however, wasn't what I always wanted to do. As doctors working towards specialist qualifications, we rotate through many different areas of medicine to round out our skills and expose us to many possible career pathways. I was desperate to be an orthopaedic or plastic surgeon, specialising in hand surgery. My mum has a dreadful form of arthritis and had her first hip replacement at 40; I was determined to cure her disease. As a kind of 'trade-off' for a rotation in orthopaedic surgery, I had to spend time in cardiothoracic surgery, which wasn't really my interest; however, when it came to the heart, it turned out to be love at first sight and I never left.

While it came as a surprise, it seems heart surgery might always have been on the cards for me. When my parents moved out of our family home, Mum rediscovered all our childhood keepsakes. Among the first-place running ribbons (my brother's) and the participation ribbons (mine) was my Grade 3 diary. I had no recollection of it, but on the page entitled 'When I grow up…', I had written, 'I want to be a heart surgeon and finish the work of Dr Victor Chang'. Dr Chang was a Sydney cardiac surgeon and one of the first to perform a heart transplant in Australia. He was shot dead in 1991, before he could complete his goal of making a durable artificial heart. I certainly had lofty aspirations for an eight-year-old.

I remember seeing Dr Chang on TV, talking about how he was making a reliable mechanical heart to cope with the shortage of donor hearts for transplant. It seemed so unreal, like science fiction. I remember Fiona Coote, the youngest Australian recipient of two heart transplants, who needed the surgery after a virus weakened her own. Other kids wanted to be ballerinas or police officers, but Chang inspired me much more than the daintiest dancer or prettiest princess. It seemed ironic that I had forgotten all of this for so many years, yet still somehow found my way to heart surgery.

There is something breathtaking the first time you see a heart on display. The sternum is divided and pulled back with a retractor, exposing the vital organ beneath it. Even as we invade its space in the chest cavity, it beats. When you touch a beating heart and feel every contraction pumping blood around the body to every vital organ, there is something magical about it. Surgeons can stop a heart to operate on it and then, when normality is restored at the completion of the operation, the heart works. It just goes back to doing its job, hopefully better than when we rudely interrupted its day.

Despite its resilience, which I adore, the heart is delicate. Every heart is different in some way, with minor variations on a theme.

One of the first transplants I ever saw was in a woman who had been born with a rare but very serious type of congenital heart defect. She was receiving a heart–lung transplant, which is one of the least commonly performed types of transplants. I cannot explain what it's like to look down and see an empty chest. When the amazing gift of the new donor organs are implanted and they start working, it's like magic or science fiction. Twelve years down the track from that day, that magic never gets old.

I still recall an early experience of meeting a lung transplant patient. I saw him in the intensive care unit two days after his surgery. I asked him how he felt. He just looked at me and said, 'You have no idea how good it feels to breathe'. That was the moment I knew that the chest and its magical organs had ensnared me and nothing would be able to replicate the fascination I felt. Coupling the beautiful science of the heart with the incredible fortune of being allowed into people's lives when they are at their most vulnerable, facing their biggest challenge and, hopefully, biggest triumph, is essentially why I love my job.

I've gone from wide-eyed and naïve young doctor to wide-eyed and less naïve slightly older doctor. Rather than holding retractors or quietly observing the heart and those who work on it, my station has been upgraded. Becoming a surgeon is something like an apprenticeship, albeit a long one. Now, I am the 'fancy plumber', as one of my mentors used to say, restoring blood flow to sick hearts and, hopefully, changing lives along the way. Sometimes, I forget the gravity of what my colleagues and I do for a living; I get lost in the routine in my job and it's not until I sit down and think about it that I remember how spectacular it truly is.

It is a big deal. A huge deal, if you will. It's incredibly cool, yet incredibly serious at the same time. Heart surgeons spend a lot of time performing coronary artery surgery, sewing together vessels that are 1 to 2 millimetres wide with a thread called a suture, not too much thicker than a human hair. We cut into the heart at just the right spot to access a diseased valve and repair it or replace it with a new one. We replumb hearts that weren't plumbed right to begin with, or make special burns in the heart muscle to direct the electricity of the heart the right way, so that it can't beat irregularly or too quickly. Often to do all of this, we stop the heart, connecting the patient to a heart–lung bypass machine, which does the work of the heart and lungs while the patient's own stay still for their surgery. This machine is run under the watchful eye of a perfusionist, a scientist who controls every part of the circulation by managing the heart–lung machine, the patient's life support.

It's a cast of thousands when it comes to heart surgery. Aside from the surgical team, which might consist of two or three surgeons, two anaesthetists and two or three nurses, all of whom are working together to perform the operation, the team extends beyond that. From the first time a patient comes into the hospital to the day they leave, there is a huge team of specialist doctors, nurses and allied health professionals, all guiding the patient and their family towards a full recovery.

The heart in all its glory

To convey what it is I love about the heart – this beautiful organ that has fascinated artists and scientists alike – I need to explain what goes on inside our chests. The heart is one of the earliest organs to form in a developing foetus. At four weeks the foetus has a very primitive four-chambered heart that starts beating. The size of an acorn or maybe a gumnut, it is tiny, yet carries so much responsibility. As the foetus develops and grows, the heart gets increasingly complicated and grows to the point that after birth, as it beats, it can sustain life. It never stops beating until the day we die.

Make a fist. That fist is roughly the size of your heart. Now think back to that gumnut – how amazing to think what a long way your heart has come. The human heart is divided into a left side and right side. Each side has two chambers: an atrium and a ventricle. So, we have a **left atrium**, **right atrium**, **left ventricle** and **right ventricle**. The heart sits in a fibrous sac called the **pericardium**, which lives directly behind the **sternum** (breastbone) and slightly to the left. It nestles into the left lung particularly, but is almost surrounded by the lungs.

The right side of the heart has two big responsibilities. The right atrium receives oxygen-poor blood from the body; this blood has fed all the hungry tissues that make up skin, bone, muscle, gut or liver. From the right atrium, blood travels through the **tricuspid valve** to the right ventricle. The right ventricle squeezes down tight and forces blood through the **pulmonary valve** and out of the **pulmonary artery**. This is its first big job: the blood travels here through the lungs to be replenished with oxygen and to expel carbon dioxide that we will eventually breathe out.

The second responsibility is for the right ventricle to provide momentum for the newly oxygenated blood to leave the lungs and travel to the left atrium via **pulmonary veins**. The left atrium drains its fresh blood through the **mitral valve** to the left ventricle. Things then get muscly. The left ventricle is like the body builder of the heart: thicker and with more muscle than the right and, when it contracts, it forces blood out at speeds of two metres per second through the **aortic valve** and into the **aorta**. The aorta is the main blood vessel of the heart and takes blood all over the body to feed the tissues that make our bodies sleep, digest, run, think, have children, sing... you name it.

A couple of other important parts help the heart do its job. The **coronary arteries** are incredibly important. The heart is, essentially, a big bag of muscle and, to do its job, muscle needs nutrients, especially oxygen and glucose. The coronary arteries deliver blood to the whole heart through an intricate network, ensuring every heart cell receives precious blood. There are three main coronary arteries: the left main coronary artery, which splits into the left circumflex artery; the left interventricular artery; and the third branch, which is the right coronary artery. When a blockage or an interruption to blood supply occurs, a **heart attack** strikes.

The other important part of the heart is its electrical system, not dissimilar to the wiring in your house. As I'm sure you've noticed, our hearts beat without being told. Lucky that, or getting distracted could be catastrophic! The wiring of the heart is called the **conduction system** and allows the electricity that fires the various parts of the heart muscle to operate in order and at a rate that is right for the body.

When the heart beats, it beats in beautiful synchrony. Blood moves from the atrium on each side into the ventricles: the atria (plural of atrium) contract and squeeze the last remaining bit of blood to the ventricles. To expel blood from the ventricles to the lungs and the body, the muscle fibres of the ventricles squeeze so forcefully that they force open the pulmonary valve and aortic valve and blood rushes out of each of these great vessels. The muscles of the ventricles don't just clamp down, but rather squeeze in a predictable pattern. The muscle fibres are arranged in a kind of spiral around the cavity of the ventricles, so that when they squeeze it's like wringing every last drop of liquid out of a cloth. When I think of the heart's amazing little details I'm in awe of the cleverness of its finer points. Even after years of evolution it is astounding that we've wound up with such a finely tuned machine.

Every day the average human heart beats at around 70 beats a minute, or 100,000 beats per day. Unlike the muscles of our arms and legs, it doesn't tire, it doesn't need a rest and it doesn't fatigue. Imagine doing 100,000 bicep curls in a day – we couldn't. Those muscles would fatigue and tire quickly, leaving us with very sore arms. The heart is very clever though, and is not set at just one rate. When you exercise your heart might beat up to 190 times per minute or more; and when you sleep – so your body is using less energy – your heart might slow to 40 beats a minute overnight. Over a lifetime this will add up to over three trillion beats.

The heart is like a machine or an appliance that you 'set and forget'. It goes as long as it has a blood supply. It doesn't need the brain to tell it to beat, how fast or when. The heart muscle cells are so incredibly clever that, as long as blood brings nutrients such as oxygen, glucose and fatty acids, the heart muscle cells beat rhythmically. And they all do it together in unison as an efficient and coordinated pump.

The functions of the heart and the way it works – from its overall pumping ability, to those processes that can only be seen with powerful microscopes – range from simple to brilliantly complex. However, when we think of how the heart just works – perfectly, beautifully and intelligently for our whole lives – it is nothing short of extraordinary.

When something goes wrong

Although finely tuned, the heart is prone to problems just like any machine. Some of these we are born with, some are destined in our genes, and some are problems that develop over a lifetime of food, exercise and smoking choices that upset its delicate balance.

A heart attack is its most common problem. A heart attack happens when one of the coronary arteries develops a blockage. These blockages tend to happen over time, as the vessels respond to factors such as the fats and sugars we eat, cigarette smoke or a change in response to our genes, our gender or our blood pressure. The walls of the coronary arteries become clogged and narrowed by plaque called **atheroma**. When they are completely clogged, usually by a clot on top of the plaque, the area of heart muscle they are supplying either dies or sometimes becomes stunned. The longer the blockage is there, the more severe the damage to the muscle, and the pumping action of the heart can be seriously impaired. **Angina,** when the narrowed coronary vessels can't provide a good blood supply, is similar to a heart attack but without the same severity. These two diseases are often lumped together as **heart disease**. Heart disease, specifically of the coronary arteries, is the leading cause of death for men and women in most developed countries, including Australia, the United States and the United Kingdom.

In these developed countries heart disease kills three times as many women as breast cancer, yet most of us don't know that. We still think of it as a man's disease: something affecting our fathers, uncles, brothers or husbands. The Heart Foundation has discovered that only three out of 10 women feel that heart disease is something they have to be personally worried about.

What's even scarier is that over 90 per cent of Australian women have at least one risk factor for heart disease; many have more. These are often risks we can do something about, such as smoking or high blood pressure. Women's heart disease is actually quite different to heart disease that afflicts men. Women have very different symptoms, such as tiredness or shortness of breath doing something that used to be easy. Blockages form differently in a woman's heart, with its smaller blood vessels and the protection of oestrogen, so the disease and the symptoms are different. In fact, scientists and doctors are still trying to work out how different treatments affect women's hearts when compared to men's.

The **valves** of the heart are highly specialised structures that ensure that blood flows in the right direction around the heart and out into the body. Normal heart valves are beautiful: they are thin and nearly translucent and look somewhat like a parachute. When blood flows past them, after a period of time, they drift shut. Blood going in the wrong direction battles like someone walking up a down escalator – it's hard work. When blood goes backwards, the extra blood that is hanging around the heart, rather than starting its journey around the body, makes the heart work extra hard. When this happens, we say that a valve has **regurgitation**. A valve can become very narrowed, sometimes less than half its normal size, which again makes the heart work a lot harder to pump blood forwards. This is called **stenosis** and sometimes happens as we age and our heart valves develop wear and tear; sometimes it's because of disease, such as rheumatic fever or an infection of the heart valve.

Sometimes a heart has a disease specific to its muscle and muscle cells. We call this **cardiomyopathy**, derived from the Latin meaning 'heart muscle disease'. Many different conditions can lead to this common end point of damaged muscle, including viral infection, heart attack or genetics, and sometimes we don't know for sure which. A proportion of these patients will go on to develop **heart failure**, when the pumping ability of the heart is severely impaired and it is unable to send enough blood to allow the body to do its job. These people can be so sick that even simple tasks, such as getting dressed or walking to the letterbox, are just not doable. Some of these patients will go on to require heart transplants.

Not every disease of the heart muscle is acquired over a lifetime. Some children are born with heart problems, known as **congenital heart disease.** Children whose hearts don't quite follow the usual pattern of development and growth in the womb are born with a wide range of heart defects, including holes in the heart called **atrial** or **ventricular septal defects**. Some children are born with heart defects that are very complex; they can be extremely unwell and must undergo surgery in the first few days of life. This is the most common form of birth defect, with one in 100 babies born with a heart defect; a third of these children require at least one surgery to fix their heart.

Today we know so much fascinating information about the heart and yet what we learn tomorrow could turn that on its head. That goes for every part of our bodies – we are always learning. Not long ago we didn't even know about DNA; now it's part of everyday conversation and a regular plotline on TV shows. Our knowledge about the heart is the same: growing all the time.

chapter 1
CAN YOU DIE OF A BROKEN HEART?

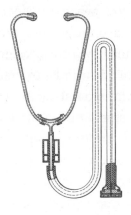

**Stab the body and it heals, but injure
the heart and the wound lasts a lifetime**
MINEKO IWASAKI, JAPANESE BUSINESSWOMAN,
AUTHOR AND FORMER GEIKO

Think of the first time you had your heart broken. It might have been last week or it might have been years ago. Most of us have experienced heartbreak and most of us have been unlucky enough to experience it more than once. The emotional insult of losing someone, whether it be the end of your first love affair, or the death of someone close to you, is hard enough. When you think about your heartbreak, it's not just emotional pain.

When you're heartbroken, your heart may actually feel hurt. Your chest feels tight or sore. Some people describe it as like a knife through the heart. It's a horrible feeling and, as your chest aches for the person you have lost, you truly wonder if you will be able to go on without them. Your family and friends tell you that life will get better and your heart will heal. Your heart mostly does heal, although it feels bruised and battered, and you do find the strength to go on. You might even find that you get stronger.

The connection between the mind and physical health has been debated for a long time. You don't have to look far to be told how the power of positive thought can change your whole life, including your physical health. Through thoughts of healing, it is said the human body can battle disease. We tell people with illnesses, such as cancer and heart disease, to 'fight' in their minds, to visualise an army of tiny soldiers who bravely march into battle. A frequent debate in the news is the link between stress and ailments like these. Heartbreak is one of the most powerful emotions we feel. When your heart is shattered into a million pieces, you feel like you may just expire. The question is, can you? Can you really die of a broken heart?

In 2016 the actress Carrie Fisher passed away, leaving hordes of *Star Wars* fans surprised and saddened. A day later her mother, Debbie Reynolds, died of a stroke. Some say Debbie's heart and body simply gave out. Desperately bereft without her daughter, Debbie 'died of a broken heart'. The press reported that the day after Carrie died her mother just asked to be with her daughter. It's a bittersweet kind of heartbreak.

The Japanese fishing pot

Medically speaking, broken heart syndrome is real. Its medical name is **takotsubo cardiomyopathy,** or stress-induced cardiomyopathy. The syndrome is similar to a heart attack: the body's emotions cause the release of huge amounts of hormones that lead the coronary arteries to spasm and squeeze down, limiting vital blood supply to the precious heart muscle cells. When heart muscle cells are damaged, they don't pump well.

Takotsubo is the name given to a kind of squid-fishing pot used by Japanese fishermen. The pot or trap has a very distinct shape with a narrow neck and a base that balloons out. When someone has takotsubo, this is how their heart looks. The narrow neck of the heart pumps and squeezes well, but the bottom (apex) of the left ventricle is the sick heart muscle that doesn't pump, so it balloons out.

What causes takotsubo, what hormones are involved and how it is best treated are still being studied. Broken heart syndrome got its name when doctors noticed it often occurred in women who had received some sort of terrible news, usually following the death of a loved one. In fact, one of the earlier cases involved a woman who came to a top-shelf hospital in Massachusetts in the early 1990s. She described the classic chest pain that everyone, including doctors, associates with heart attacks. When they performed a test to look at her coronary arteries, they expected to see blockages that would account for her heart attack. There were none, but it was then revealed that her teenage son had committed suicide that day. It would be years before the term takotsubo would be used and the connection between the mind and the heart would be viewed by medical professionals as more than just folklore.

A feminine issue?

Women are much more likely to be affected by broken heart syndrome. Up to 90 per cent of patients with this disease are female; the remaining 10 per cent of male patients tend to be 'shocked' by a physical, rather than emotional, trauma, such as being in a fight. In some cases the 'shock' has been associated with amphetamine use, which, just like emotional stress or physical trauma, floods the body's organs with hormones that are supposed to help us face an adversary or retreat (a fight-or-flight response). To muddy the waters, the symptoms people present with are very similar to a typical heart attack.

In February 2011 the New Zealand city of Christchurch experienced a severe earthquake. Christchurch is the country's second largest city with a population of around 340,000. The 6.3 magnitude quake struck just after lunchtime. In addition to the loss of 185 lives in the earthquake and huge damage to the city, the number of people who presented at hospital with heart issues rose sharply. In the four days that followed, 21 people were diagnosed with takotsubo or stress-induced cardiomyopathy. To put that into perspective, we normally see a few of these cases in an entire year.

As expected from what we already know of this disease, the 21 were all female. Most of them were otherwise well: they weren't smokers or diabetics, nor did they have high blood pressure, which most of us know as typical risk factors for heart disease. A year after the quake all the women were alive and well. Some people succumb to their condition while others, receiving care to support the heart, recover well.

Fight or flight

The bodies of those with broken heart syndrome are pumping out large amounts of hormones, such as adrenaline, noradrenaline and dopamine. Adrenaline is a hormone produced by the adrenal glands and by some nerve cells in the body. It's what causes your heart to beat fast and your pupils to dilate as if you're ready for a fight, which is exactly what adrenaline exists for – the fight-or-flight response that harks back to our days of running from sabre-toothed tigers. It makes our hearts pump faster, pushes up our blood pressure and makes us sweat. Any scary or emotionally overwhelming experience can result in the body pumping out adrenaline.

Medical research is still trying to work out the intricacies of takotsubo, but we do know the likely reason for the reaction comes down to hormones. The brain is shocked emotionally and a particular primitive part of the brain called the hypothalamus kicks things off. It starts telling the pituitary and adrenal glands and the nerves of the autonomic nervous system to pump out a lot of adrenaline. The adrenaline causes the blood vessels of the heart to squeeze down, almost as if they were afraid. This is particularly noticeable in the smaller blood vessels of the heart which squeeze down, effectively shutting down blood supply to the heart muscle cells. As the blood vessels all squeeze down, blood pressure skyrockets and the heart has to pump extra hard against the added blood pressure, which makes the heart sick.

If we take a biopsy of heart muscle tissue from a heart with takotsubo, we can use a microscope to see what happens to the cells. The huge rush of adrenaline and other stress hormones damages the specialised proteins inside the cells; these proteins act as machinery for the cells to contract and cause the heart to pump. Some studies have shown that the various parts of the muscle cells including the mitochondria (the parts of a cell that deliver power to that cell) are damaged. Takotsubo heart cells experience widespread damage, probably from a kind of internal overdose of adrenaline.

This is where the heart is pretty cool, but also pretty vulnerable. Heart muscle cells are amazing. To squeeze and pump, heart muscle cells need blood, which has glucose and oxygen for energy and electrolytes like calcium, potassium and sodium, to move in and out of the cell. The blood also takes away waste products, such as carbon dioxide. Once you give the heart muscle cells the energy they need and remove the waste products they don't, they contract and shorten. When you have a whole heart worth of muscle cells getting blood, you have a heart that pumps with every beat. However, take away this blood delivery and removal system, and the heart muscle cells go out to lunch. Take it away for long enough and those cells can die. With enough cardiac muscle damage you will have a heart that isn't interested in pumping.

The weaker sex?

As much as society may like to pin takotsubo on women because they're perceived as more emotional, it's probably not quite that straightforward. In fact, many other cellular processes, body signals and hormones are responsible here, and medical science is still trying to work them out. Factors such as the way the body handles fatty acids or glucose are at play. Fatty acids and glucose provide energy for cells to perform their basic processes, such as moving, making protein or even growing and dividing. In sick cells, such as in takotsubo, there could be a problem with the muscle cell's ability to effectively use this energy source.

Oestrogen protects the heart, so when oestrogen starts to decline in menopause, the heart may be more vulnerable, particularly the blood vessels of the heart, which can be extra reactive. This may account for the fact that women are afflicted by takotsubo more than men. But we don't yet fully understand why some people get this, or what level of stress will start the process.

A heart affected by takotsubo cardiomyopathy can get very sick. And that in turn can make its owner very sick. There's no actual cure. We use treatments that are broadly termed 'supportive care': medicines that take the strain off the sick heart; medicines that oppose the ill effects of these adrenaline-type hormones; and medicines that relax blood vessels to make the heart's job a little easier. Sicker patients might need medicines to help the heart pump or raise the blood pressure so that all the other vital organs receive blood. Most people with takotsubo make a perfectly fine recovery, as the heart recovers from the stress hormone storm. Some do not, and some even die of their broken heart.

I just can't beat without you

One Friday we operated on a gentleman who could be described as 'a character'. He had lived a phenomenally interesting life and was widowed but in a de facto relationship with a wonderfully free-spirited woman. They met online when they were both 70 years old, starting a long-distance relationship and eventually moving to the same city to be together. They loved life and it was evident they loved each other. They were comfortable and cheeky together and had a social life that would make most 30-somethings feel like hermits. He had been sick, which dulled his exuberance, and she had been worried. Despite his protestations that he wasn't that sick, she knew when he came home from his daily walk and couldn't breathe well. She forced him into an ambulance. (It's often women who forcibly make their partners use an ambulance!) He had developed a bad infection around his lung and needed surgery to relieve the infection, reinflate the lung and fix his breathing.

He didn't make it. The infection was severe and at 82 his fragile body had been overwhelmed. His sparkle and liveliness, his fitness, even their wonderful life and love together couldn't outsmart the infection and the stress of a big surgery.

That evening will always be stuck in my mind. I remember calling his partner, June, to break the bad news. She immediately made her way into the hospital. I went to do part of my job I hate most – telling the family of patients who didn't make it what had happened and how incredibly sorry I was. It was getting late and although it had been a long week, my registrar and I sat with June and a nurse for over an hour. Initially because we didn't want her to be alone while she waited for her daughter to arrive, but then for another reason altogether: we sat to listen.

June told us all about their life: how they had met, the movies they loved, their children from their previous marriages and how she used to tease him incessantly because he was Scottish and she was English. She told us about the blues band they had seen at the local pub only two weeks earlier, and how their dogs tried to steal the bed sheets. I sat there, transfixed at this story because it touched my heart so much. They were so in love and so full of life. It was so beautiful and her face was showing the extraordinary happiness they brought one another. She wept and said, 'I just can't believe he's gone, how am I ever supposed to be without him?' I was beginning to wonder the same thing. I don't know what happened to June but I hope that her heart was strong enough to survive.

The bereaved soul

Not uncommonly, we read of tales of spouses who die within days or weeks of one another. Don and Maxine Simpson met in 1952 and married not long after. They were inseparable, doing everything together. Maxine died at the age of 87 and four hours later Don slipped away too. It is like a last gasp of true love that the two hearts can't beat apart. Not exactly broken heart syndrome, but another way of the heart giving in when our souls are hurting after bereavement.

Isn't it romantic? Doesn't that seem like the ultimate gesture of love – that your heart is so broken you simply cannot go on with it? The theme is popular in films such as *The Notebook,* in which the romance of truly being unable to live without your other half was turned into a gut-wrenching tale. I'm sure that's why when we hear stories about dying of a 'broken heart', despite being sad, it's also somehow endearing. Can two hearts be so intertwined that they simply cannot beat without the other? Hundreds of years ago, before Leonardo da Vinci made his beautiful drawings of the heart, scholars actually did believe that the heart was the centre of the soul.

I look inside hearts pretty regularly these days and I'm yet to locate a soul, but I am sure of one thing... The heart may not be the centre or the origin of the soul or our emotions, but it is most definitely affected by them. The chest is the place we often feel emotions most strongly. It feels that dull ache when we've lost someone, the tightness of anxiety, or the lightness of love or elation. If we concentrate, we can feel our hearts skip along when we're happy or thunder when we're scared. We even sometimes feel that our hearts skip a beat at the sight of the love of our life. While some of these feelings are cultural sayings, some are the body's reaction to our emotions.

It may seem an obvious statement, but bereavement is as bad for your body as it is for your soul. If you have ever lost anyone, you'll know that incredible cloud of grief that covers everything you think and do. I see bereavement in many forms. Sometimes it's stoic and strong. Some people are very matter-of-fact, while others look on the bright side by acknowledging their loved one is at peace or with a special family member. Some just cry, and others are beyond consolation. I once had a table thrown at me when delivering bad news. No judgement there: grief is a nasty piece of work.

Presumably following the anecdotes of grandmas and grandpas who died within a short space of time, studies have now been done into death by broken heart. Not surprisingly, it seems to be a real phenomenon. Researchers have looked at many different couples over many years to work out what happens to that bereaved partner when they find themselves without their true love. It is done in a scientific manner by studying someone who has lost a partner and comparing them with someone of a similar age who hasn't lost a partner. This is a scientific way of reducing confounding factors. We want to be sure the effect we're seeing is due to bereavement, rather than some other factor that messes up the result, in this case age.

What we see is this: regardless of the group we look at, men or women, husbands or wives, even parents, there is a trend to suggest that the risk of dying is higher after the loss of someone important and close to you. This risk seems to be highest in older people (seventies or older) and in those who have experienced that loss recently, within 30 days. One study even showed that on the first day after losing someone, the risk of having a heart attack is 16 times greater than normal. Some studies report a 66-fold increase in the death of widowers in the first 30 days. Men are more likely to die soon after their partners. What creates this skew in the sexes? Possibly it's because when they've lost their partner many men have also lost their sole confidante (whereas women are more likely to have a circle of friends they confide in). It could also relate to the fact that it is often the woman who oversees the man's health: when she is gone, there is nobody to nag him to take care of himself anymore.

Studies have shown that spouses and parents of a person who has committed suicide have an increased risk of death, specifically by suicide. This group warrants very special attention and, as healthcare professionals or simply as family and friends of the bereaved, we should be ready to offer any help we can give them. The loss of someone who ended their own life doesn't just stress the workings of the body, but creates an extremely dark place for these people; their hearts and souls often just can't take it.

The stress of loss

Studies have looked at the way the body responds to grief. Cortisol is a great stress hormone; it's made by two little glands called the adrenals, which sit on top of your kidneys in the abdomen. When you're feeling stressed, a part of your brain called the hypothalamus sends signals to the adrenal glands to release cortisol and the cortisol mobilises your body for a fight. It starts by pumping glucose from storage houses such as your liver and muscle cells to provide energy to run away. Cortisol also alters your immune system. It's partly good, because it stops your body going too crazy with inflammation, which can sometimes cause disease, but it also can reduce your body's ability to fight off infection. In people who have lost someone close to them, cortisol levels remain high for up to six months – so six months of not being able to fight infection. Cortisol also ruins energy stores, and can prevent wounds healing. So, while cortisol is a necessary part of the way our bodies deal with stress, when we flog ourselves with it for too long it can actually make us sick.

During times of grief your brain can ruin your sleep, which then affects your immune system and reduces your ability to fight off many types of disease. The heart is particularly vulnerable in times of grief – people who are grieving have higher heart rates, higher blood pressure and increases in funny heart rhythms, all of which place an enormous stress on the heart. Even their blood is more prone to clotting, which means that people who are grieving are more liable to clogged-up arteries, particularly in hearts that might already have disease.

Many of the ways our bodies respond to threats such as stress, infection or injury are important and have evolved over many years to save lives. But they can also create mischief, especially when they're left unchecked. The poor old heart is stuck at the centre of this cascade of hormones and blood pressure changes and can really suffer. So, if someone is already a little vulnerable to a heart problem, say because of age or gender, and they lose their partner, then they can be – in a very real sense – at risk of dying from a broken heart.

Breaking up and breaking hearts

Here's a personal tale for you. My own biggest relationship heart-break very nearly broke me. As you would expect, I spent a lot of time crying, talking, crying again and then talking some more to my friends. It was a horrible time – not only had I lost my partner and best friend, but I also felt I had lost all those happy memories we had shared. They were tainted by this new pain. I remember talking to a friend about this and how I felt so sad to have lost those beautiful stories. Somehow, we got talking about how, when someone you love dies, those memories may not be quite so tainted. They continue to be beautiful and happy, as they always were.

Like a lot of people in that situation, my heart was broken but my body was not far behind. I didn't sleep; I couldn't sleep. I had *Mad Men* on repeat on my laptop so that if I did happen to nod off, when I woke up, I wouldn't be alone – Don Draper and his misfit colleagues would be there to greet me. My appetite was non-existent and I became thin and gaunt. My clothes hung off me and my hair was lank. My body was undernourished and running on adrenaline. My heart hurt so badly that it was destroying the rest of me in the process.

While separation, divorce or losing your high-school boyfriend are, of course, not the same as watching your soulmate die, they still give a massive beating to your mind and body. Medical science has devised ways to take pictures of the brain by magnetic resonance imaging (MRI). Even better, we can use a specific form of functional MRI to light up areas of the brain that are particularly active, so we can see in the images which areas are working overtime and which are chilling out. When it comes to breaking up, the brain is not happy about it. One great, if slightly mean, study showed photos of their ex-partners to people who had recently suffered a breakup. What did they find? The parts of the brain that detect pain lit up like crazy. So, you are genuinely in pain when your happy-ever-after turns sour.

People are pretty quick to point out that divorce is common these days, and one of the more stressful life events that can happen. This is hardly surprising when you consider it isn't just losing a relationship and a partner, but perhaps children, property, pets and even favourite belongings. Plus, divorce is a potentially expensive venture. Relationship breakups can create stress on top of stress and, as we know when it comes to bereavement, stress is not great for you.

Quite a few people have looked at how divorce impacts specifically on the heart. Women going through divorce seem to be prone to having their hearts literally broken. If we look at men and women after divorce, women's health takes more of a hit; men remarry more often and sooner, which may help their emotional and physical health. Women are generally more emotionally and financially hurt in a marriage breakdown, which adds a whole bunch of pain to an already rubbish situation. When it comes to men's health after divorce, it seems that, once again, not having someone around to nag them to eat well and drink less is a bad thing for their health. Keep that in mind if you're a woman who has been accused of nagging: it's for the good of their health.

For women who are divorced, the risk of a heart attack is between 1.29 to 1.39 times higher than for women who are continuously married. For men, the figures are similar, with the risk of heart attack for divorcees 1.38 times greater than for their married counterparts. What is different, though, is that when men remarry that risk drops back down to a similar level to that of their continuously married mates. To put this into perspective, the risks posed by divorce to a woman's heart health is on a similar level to that of high blood pressure or smoking.

Two studies have specifically looked at what happens to blood pressure when someone is getting divorced or thinking about their divorce. These studies showed a big jump in the blood pressure of these heartbroken individuals. Once again, this was more pronounced for women than men. High blood pressure puts incredible stress on the heart and blood vessels. While much is made of the traditional risks for heart problems, such as smoking and diet, divorce is emerging as the way to really break your heart. A US study of more than 16,000 patients found a scary trend: for both men and women divorce increases the risk of having a heart attack; however, for women that risk is even higher, especially for women who are currently divorced. Now here's when things get a little unfair for the ladies. If you remarry, your risk of a heart attack doesn't lower. For the blokes, however, the risk goes down a little. And, unsurprisingly, the more divorces you have the worse it is for your heart.

Being happily, continuously married is a pretty good way to avoid heartbreak on all fronts. Women who are married seem to have their hearts well looked after because they smoke less and exercise more. When we take into account all the factors that can make you more or less healthy – such as where you live and how much money you make – women who are married may have a similar rate of heart attacks to those who are unmarried, but they do a lot better in the long run. By doing better, I mean they are more likely to survive a heart attack and afterwards they live a better quality of life. The real advantage though is for married men, who really take the prize if they're married, because in virtually every study they do much better than single men after a heart attack.

Heart attacks are not the only problem that can be precipitated by the death of a loved one or a relationship breakup. **Atrial fibrillation** is a heart rhythm that is abnormal. Rather than contracting regularly and evenly, the atria fibrillate, meaning that they shake and contract in an uncoordinated fashion. Atrial fibrillation is one of the most common heart problems and can lead to further issues, including heart failure or clots forming in the uncoordinated areas of the atrium, which can then move to the brain, blocking off blood supply and causing a stroke.

If you lose a partner, your risk of developing atrial fibrillation is around 1.5 times that of the general population. This is more pronounced in younger people and that risk remains elevated for around one year after your partner dies. Much like heart attacks or other health problems such as infection or trauma, the body responds to stress through activation of its nerves and hormone systems (including adrenaline and the sympathetic nervous system). That in itself can cause the heart to flick into atrial fibrillation.

The ways in which the heart can be more than just emotionally battered by a breakup are similar to the symptoms that can appear when a spouse dies. Hormones such as cortisol, which cause problems with sleep and blood pressure, are released when you are told that 'it's not you; it's me'. And it seems those processes that cause physical problems in our bodies don't just hang around until we're over the heartbreak: they seem to cause health issues that are, to some degree, sustained. Depressing, right? Becoming a cat lady might be looking pretty attractive about now.

So can you die of a broken heart?

In short, yes you can. From the direct toxic effects of adrenaline in an acutely stressful situation, to the physical symptoms of having your heart broken, the mind and heart are truly connected. However, the less straightforward answer is that while having a broken heart will not always kill you, it certainly is not good for your physical wellbeing. While your body is trying to be helpful by setting off a cascade of hormones and nervous system responses to be ready to fight for your survival, these effects can actually hurt your heart when they hang around for too long. The tough thing about life is that we truly cannot avoid the rough times. So is there a way to protect yourself?

Well, I suppose you could avoid love altogether, but where is the fun in that? We know that being married or in a relationship is protective, and not just for health. After all, when love is around, isn't life wonderful? It seems that most of the population is more than happy to risk it for the glorious rewards. While rough times can be guaranteed, building a resilient body and mind is like taking out an insurance policy for your wellbeing.

chapter 2
STRESSED-OUT HEARTS

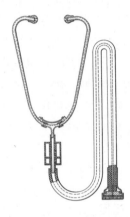

Reality is the leading cause of stress
LILY TOMLIN, WRITER, COMEDIAN AND ACTOR

'You'll give yourself a heart attack!' my mum would say to my dad when I was small and he was upset about something. My dad had a temper, often brought on by my brother and me getting up to no good. After Dad had shown us the error of our ways, Mum would add the cherry on top by detailing how much stress he was under at work and how unfair it was that he had to have stress at home too. We were going to 'give him a heart attack'.

Even as a know-it-all eight-year-old, I had my doubts about Mum's correlation of heart attacks with our causing trouble on our BMX bikes. It seemed so melodramatic. However, I certainly didn't want to be the cause of Dad keeling over. It was a common thing in those days to be told not to stress someone who is sick – it was bad for their body or their heart or their headache. Being stressed and frazzled was always explained by the adults around me as such a drain on the body that I started to think it must be true.

The physiology of stress

We all feel stress from time to time; some of us more often than others, and some more deeply than others. Take a moment to think back to the last time you were stressed. Maybe it was at work, maybe you were waiting in a queue somewhere, or getting stuck at every red traffic light when you were already running late. Picture that situation as if it were happening to you right now. Think about how your body feels. Notice your heartbeat. Do you feel tightness in your chest? Perhaps you're getting a headache. Your emotions at the time were probably those we associate with stress, such as anger, panic, fear, frustration, embarrassment or other unpleasant sensations. Despite that emotion being a function of your brain, your personality and how you see the world, your physical body does not escape that feeling.

Most of the time when I look at a heart, its owner is under deep anaesthetic. But before they go off to sleep for their surgery that person is hooked up to many different monitors to measure heart rate, blood pressure and even brain waves. I'm on the other side of the operating table but I can only imagine the incredible amount of stress people feel when they are wheeled into that theatre for the huge event ahead.

I have watched the heartbeats and blood pressure of my patients reflected in the monitors as they go off to sleep for their surgery. Even if they didn't say, we can tell those who are more anxious than others. The green lines of their heart rates fill the screen faster; the red line of blood pressure shows a higher number. Their minds and hearts sense the impending surgery and respond accordingly.

Thanks to the skill of our anaesthetists who slowly drift the patient off to sleep, their minds relax and their hearts follow suit. The green lines slow down and the blood pressure numbers, flashing in bright red, float down to a normal level. The heart breathes a sigh of relief as the stress is now out of the patient's hands and firmly in ours.

Barbara's story

I remember a particular patient who was very stressed before her surgery. Her name was Barbara and, up until a few weeks prior, she'd felt fine. Barbara was one of those women who didn't really have time to be unwell: she was a full-time carer for her husband who was quite sick. Eventually, after a fortnight of ignoring the niggles of pain in her chest, Barbara relented and saw her doctor. She was shipped off to the hospital in an ambulance – Barbara had suffered a heart attack and was now awaiting heart surgery.

Most of our patients in hospital awaiting surgery have little wires stuck on their chests connecting them to heart monitors, which can alert us to any signs of trouble. Barbara was very nervous: about her surgery, about her husband, about her future. We sat in her hospital room the night before her surgery and, as we spoke, out of the corner of my eye, I watched the heart rate climb. I saw Barbara start to perspire as her voice shook, asking questions about this huge operation she was about to have. Tears welled up in her eyes and she told me several times just how scared she was.

As the stress climbed, her heart rate and blood pressure continued to climb. Barbara stopped mid-sentence and said to me, 'I really don't feel that well'. The anxiety and emotional stress of her illness and her operation had put very real physical stress on her heart. We stopped our consultation and started doing all the things we do to rescue sick hearts: giving painkillers and the medicines that relax the tightened blood vessels and those that slow the heart.

39

They were all aimed at directly opposing the dangerous effects of stress being forced upon Barbara's vulnerable heart. She settled her mind and her heart soon followed.

We gingerly finished the conversation and, as I left the room, Barbara launched herself at me, hugging me tightly and crying, asking us all to take extra special care of her. Barbara's operation went extremely well and she was back with her husband only five days later. Her very understandable emotional stress, though, put all that pressure on her heart, showing just how interconnected our minds and bodies can be.

Stress of mind and body

When I feel stressed, my shoulders tense and rise up towards my ears. My jaw tenses and my teeth grind on each other. My brow furrows and, if this stress persists for long enough, the tensing of my face and jaw muscles gives me a headache. I also get a feeling of tightness in my chest, as if someone is pushing directly on the centre of my chest and my breathing is shallow. When I focus on my heart, it's beating quite quickly and forcefully, almost as if it's trying to expel those negative emotions from itself. Once the stress goes away, I feel physically tired and drained, a little like I've run a marathon.

When you imagine or experience those emotions and then take note of what your body physically experiences, it becomes clear that emotional stress can affect or even harm your physical wellbeing. Even before medicine acknowledged the ill effects of the stressors of life, doctors and nurses understood that you shouldn't fatigue an already worn-out and sick body with any kind of stress. The reasoning wasn't quite there, or wasn't very accurate, but there was an inkling that burdening someone who had just had a heart attack was not the right thing to do. People who had suffered a heart attack were placed on bed rest and their families whispered the problems of the world or of the patient among themselves, desperate to avoid upsetting the recovering heart.

For many years, certain personality types were thought to be at risk for heart disease. Even as far back as the 1930s, doctors and researchers noted that patients who had been treated for a psychiatric illness had higher rates of death due to heart disease than those who had not. Those findings were repeated in other studies of mental illness, including depression and bipolar disorder. Since those observations were made, personality style became linked to heart disease, with emotions such as anger and hostility or tendencies to hopelessness becoming associated with higher risk of heart attack or heart disease.

Since the 1930s, stress has been studied extensively as a nasty little beast that attacks your health. Chronic stress, whether it occurs in childhood or adulthood, increases the risk of having heart disease by up to 60 per cent. Let's say we had 200 people of all shapes and sizes and 100 of them report that life is pretty sweet and they don't experience significant amounts of stress. In the other corner we have 100 people who find things a little harder and report significant stress. Around 30 to 50 people in the first group have heart disease; in the stressed group, that number could be as high as 60 people.

It's not just heart problems either. A large study, involving thousands of people, looked at the association of long working hours with stroke and heart attack and found the risk of stroke increased in those working longer than normal hours. Stress can cause problems with the brain, which in turn upsets the body's delicate hormonal balance and make us more prone to diseases such as diabetes.

So what constitutes the kind of stress that will make us sick? While queuing for your morning coffee is annoying, it's probably not a stress that is dangerous to your wellbeing. But work stress, loneliness, bereavement or financial strain can all have an impact on physical health. These are life's big trials and tribulations.

If stress is bad for us, shouldn't we just take care of it in whatever way we can? Smoking is apparently a great stress release, as is eating chocolate or having a drink or two. But as much as I would love to eat away my stress for the good of my heart, it doesn't work like that. You see, when we have a group of risk factors for a disease, some will cause disease very easily and consistently, others not consistently. This can be termed 'the effect'. If we look at the effect of smoking on heart disease, it's pretty high. With stress, the effect is not consistent; we don't know how strongly our own body will react.

Stress is also a necessary part of life. Without it, we can never improve and change. In some ways it's very similar to 'stressing' the body with exercise to build it up. I have to be honest, I love a bit of pressure. It focuses me and pushes me to do better. Most of us exist on a continuum of stress: too little and we get complacent or lazy, but too much means we can't physically or mentally do what's asked of us.

In the right doses, psychological stress can be helpful. If we sail through life without ever facing difficulty, we will not be able to build tools such as resilience to help us through the inevitable tough times. We need to strike a balance between so little stress that we don't develop psychological tools, and so much stress that it just weighs us down.

Heart surgery can be a tough gig – a real stress inducer. And that is just for those of us doing it, let alone the patients. Luckily, I suppose, I like stress more than most people. I once hosted a charity event where the organisers were concerned that, as a non-professional presenter, I might feel stressed in front of an audience. I remember laughing and saying, 'Well, I think I'll be fine, because nobody's going to die if I make a mistake!' Everyone laughed, but

I merely meant to illustrate that stress doesn't bother me as much as others, especially when I compare situations like that to my day job. Being relatively resilient to stress is an important attribute for working in my field. Doctors can quite literally hold life in their hands and that is a big responsibility to shoulder. I'm grateful for the trust people give me in those moments.

Even though I can shoulder stress relatively well, I can also slide down the other side of the curve of stress and productivity. I remember a particularly challenging week at work. It had begun with the death of a patient who was very unwell and probably not expected to live very long, but it still hurt me badly. The rest of the week didn't bring much relief. I operated on some of the sickest hearts and tried to do their owners justice, ensuring every hair-like stitch was placed with the utmost precision. Despite this, some of these sick people had complications in their operations and in recovering afterwards. It was a week filled with worry, serious conversations with families, serious conversations with colleagues, and long hours. On the last day of that miserable week, one of my patients became sick and had to be tested to see if his operation had worked. I remember my fears very distinctly. I wondered if I had somehow jeopardised his recovery and began to replay every minute detail of his care.

While waiting for his test results that Sunday morning, I remember thinking 'this week has been too much' – and it had. The events and long hours had exhausted my reserve and I began to feel the negative effects of stress. I was tired and grumpy, I couldn't be bothered with exercise and I certainly didn't feel I had any energy to expend on myself. My head thumped and I found myself craving sugary foods. I was starting to exhaust myself trying to keep up. Fortunately, my patient's test results were good and the operation had been successful. He made a slow but steady recovery, as did I from the week's events.

Stress: modus operandi

Stress causes issues in two different ways. Firstly, it makes us more likely to do things that aren't great for our health, such as abandoning exercise in favour of eating biscuits. Secondly, it directly hurts our body. I find this fascinating, because turning long hours into a heart attack seems like a big leap.

So, let's start with the more interesting side of the equation. Like a lot of things, testing for the effect of stress on your body is hard to do in a truly scientific fashion. It's difficult, not to mention unethical, to take a bunch of people and subject them to some form of life stress until they have heart attacks. So we have to rely on the next most scientific method and that is animal studies or observational studies. Animal studies are pretty self-explanatory. An observational study can be done without messing about with a person's life too much. We watch a group of people for an outcome, say a heart attack, while at the same time seeing who is stressed, or who smokes, or who wears red shoes, then look for an increase (or decrease) of heart disease in those subgroups. So, if we find the people wearing red shoes have more heart attacks than those who wear black shoes, then there would be a possible association or a risk that wearing red shoes is bad for your heart. It's imperfect, but sometimes it's the best research tool we have.

When it comes to stress, we can see an association between social stress and heart issues. This is interesting because, as well as being closely related to humans, monkeys and other primates have social norms and social structures just like us. Monkeys who experience social stress develop blockages of the heart arteries faster than those who are pretty chilled. They also tend to stack on fat around their midsections as the body's stress hormones, such as cortisol, are activated. Other hormones activated by stress are geared towards hanging on to so-called 'bad cholesterol', low-density lipoprotein (LDL), as well as promoting inflammation which directly damages the cells that line the blood vessels, including those around the heart.

Being constantly under the pump can make you more prone to developing **metabolic syndrome**. Metabolic syndrome is a group of illnesses or features including central adiposity (carrying extra weight around the midsection), high blood pressure, high blood glucose, high blood trigylcerides (another type of 'bad' cholesterol or fat in the blood) and low levels of the 'good' cholesterol called high-density lipoprotein (HDL). Metabolic syndrome is considered a direct precursor to heart disease and stroke because when you put all of these pieces together they attack your body to create disease.

High blood pressure directly attacks the blood vessels, heart and brain. We describe something or someone who annoys us as 'putting up our blood pressure', and it turns out that is actually true. When you're annoyed or lonely or stressed, you have increases in your blood pressure. The jury is still out as to whether these small transient increases can lead to more permanent high blood pressure. But the likelihood is that you are much more likely to have high blood pressure the more of these blips you have.

In terms of recovery after a heart attack, the chances are that your emotional state has an impact on how well you can bounce back. Feeling down is not a great thing for your sick heart. Depression is common after heart attacks, with around 20 per cent of patients having clinical depression and another quarter having milder forms of the disorder. These patients are more likely to die from their heart disease. Clinical depression is not the same as a life stress, but it does suggest that when you feel overloaded, it doesn't help the poor heart heal. Even having ongoing work stress or financial stress is not a good thing for those trying to recover.

Here's where things get even more interesting. No two people have the same reaction. If we subject two people to the same stress, say working long hours, some will thrive and others will hate it. It doesn't take much to think of someone who seems to bounce back from hardships compared to someone else who takes things to heart (pun intended). Aside from their emotional reactions, the way people's bodies react to stress by creating disease is very different. Some people hardly turn a hair; others have very quick responses in their hearts or their blood vessels that tell us they are at high risk for problems such as heart attacks.

Not only do no two people react in exactly the same way to stress, but because we can't give a measured dose of stress and watch for a response, there are also likely to be other factors that muddy the waters. This is where your reaction to stress comes into play. Is the reaction the direct effect of stress or is it the fact that you dealt with it by eating a packet of doughnuts? Chronic stress also makes it harder to exercise and, since exercise protects against heart disease, that too can play a role. It can be very hard to tease out these different aspects of causes in a complex problem such as heart disease.

Stress vs the heart: the low down

* *There is a definite increase in risk of heart disease with long-term stress.*
* *Only part of this increase can be explained by the direct effects stress has on the functioning of your body, such as hormones.*
* *Stress is probably responsible for causing heart problems by changing your body's inner workings or your behavioural response (eating, less exercise, smoking).*
* *An emotional stress can cause a major cardiac event in those who are already prone to it and upset recovery in those who have already had a heart attack.*
* *No two people have the same emotional or physical response to stress.*

Where is all this stress coming from?

It seems there is an awful lot of stress flying around these days. Everyone you speak to seems to be stressed about something. Some of the big stressors in life probably come as no surprise at all. Death of a spouse or a family member, divorce or a relationship breakdown, moving house or losing your job are some of the big-ticket items that cause upheaval. For a lot of us though, work is a huge stress-giver. People are not only working longer hours, but smart phones can mean that we are now always 'at work'.

Social media has some wonderful benefits but can actually help in creating stress, as well as reducing our ability to manage it. How often are you up late, messaging someone or scrolling through a feed and comparing your life to someone else's? We sleep less, we interact poorly and we compare more. If you're tired, your stress-fighting abilities are not at their sharpest and that can make you sicker.

Take a chill pill: mindfulness, yoga and destressing strategies

I'm sure this will come as no surprise but sometimes my life can be pretty stressful. I might say to friends that I'm feeling stressed and I'll be inundated with advice: yoga, running, attacking a punch bag or meditation have all been suggested as ways that I can destress.

I know when I feel stressed in the moment. That feeling of tightness in my chest, my teeth grinding and that horrendous headache. But the kind of stress that builds up over the longer term can sometimes be more difficult to spot. Every year at medical school I would study to the point of near exhaustion. The day exams finished every year I got flu. It was my body's way of saying that it had well and truly had enough.

Another physical sign of stress for me is that my sleep either becomes incredibly broken or I sleep too much. But it's hard to see the signs and do things that help you take care of yourself. Sometimes it's because we're too busy, or because we're in denial. I am particularly good at denial. Taking the attitude that 'this too will pass' has a role; however, blatantly ignoring a problem is not a great idea.

One of my favourite ways of alleviating stress is through mindfulness practice. The idea of mindfulness is centred on presence and observation, learning to sit with yourself physically and mentally. It's a process of paying attention to internal and external experiences, such as your breathing or the sound of cars driving by. The idea is that it's not just a skill to learn so you can sit on a pillow and chant, but a skill that can be integrated into your everyday life. You learn how to do lots of things mindfully, such as walking, eating or working.

When it comes to health benefits, mindfulness produces many stress-reducing effects that can help to ward off disease and fight existing disease. Specifically, mindfulness-based stress reduction programs can help get your body and mind in disease-fighting shape. Mindfulness can even help to alleviate symptoms such as pain. A number of studies have looked at the effect mindfulness has on managing chronic pain or depression and anxiety, and most show that the practice of mindfulness is definitely beneficial.

Stressing a sick heart is not good for the healing heart. The sick heart, though, seems to benefit from mindfulness. When patients who had heart failure (where the heart muscle is too sick to pump blood around the body) underwent training in mindfulness, they reported that their symptoms of anxiety and depression dropped. In fact, they dropped so much that over the following year, this group had less 'flare-ups' and were admitted to hospital less than those who didn't learn this skill. Just like with any other form of stress, living with a chronic disease such as heart failure makes your body work hard, firing up those fight-or-flight systems.

A stress-reduction mindfulness program is able to switch off or turn down the volume on the hormones and nerve impulses that can end up hurting an already sick heart.

There is merit to using mindfulness as a way of preventing heart disease and its accomplices such as high blood pressure. Practising mindfulness at any age reduces blood pressure and heart rate. Since having high blood pressure and a perpetually fast heart rate makes your heart work harder than it needs to, any way to reduce those two conditions can do great things for the health of your heart.

Yoga has been studied not just for its ability to produce relaxation but also its effects on the health and fitness of your heart and lungs. For those of us who like getting into downward dog, yoga can help lower blood pressure as well as improve your levels of good (HDL) and bad (LDL) cholesterol. It may even help maintain a healthy body weight. Yoga is a unique form of exercise; not only does it provide actual physical activity, but the more spiritual and mindful side of yoga practice can help manage psychological stress and alleviate anxiety.

Other forms of exercise are also very useful at helping your heart become and stay healthy. Not only does regular exercise improve your blood pressure, cholesterol and weight, it also helps elevate mood as your brain secretes chemicals that make you feel good: the so-called 'runner's high'. Exercise and being physically fit may also tone down your body-releasing stress hormones such as cortisol, helping to reduce the negative effects cortisol has on your health when it's pumped around for a long time.

Exercise is also a great way to make your blood vessels healthy – since your heart is at the centre of the blood vessels and is dependent on them to give it blood, this is incredibly important. Physical activity is amazing at improving the way blood flows. When blood flows abnormally through blood vessels, they get damaged inside; and when your blood vessels get damaged, they form plaques which eventually grow to obstruct them. When this happens in the heart, we have heart attacks.

So all around, exercise, whether it's yoga or pounding the pavement, is a two-for-the-price-of-one treatment for stress. It knocks stress on the head and makes your body physically strong and healthy to fight stress and disease.

Regardless of what you do to manage your stress, be sure to take a holistic approach with mindfulness and some sort of physical activity. Stress is neither good nor bad, but when it happens all the time, it's no good for the health of your heart or anything else. Find out what it is that makes your jaw relax or allows you to sleep better and do it.

chapter 3
'NEW' HEARTS: TRANSPLANTS AND MECHANICAL HEARTS

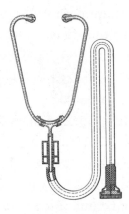

**As for you, my galvanized friend, you want a heart.
You don't know how lucky you are not to have one.
Hearts will never be practical until they can be
made unbreakable**

THE WIZARD OF OZ

It was, in fact, transplant that cemented my interest in becoming a heart surgeon. Patients who couldn't breathe, couldn't do something as simple as dressing themselves, were given a new lease of life. When they awoke from surgery, even with the tough road of rehabilitation or illness ahead, they were often immediately able to feel a change, an improvement in themselves.

Michael's story

Years ago, I met a patient called Michael. He was a shade of grey that humans shouldn't normally be. It's a colour we associate with being really, really ill. Michael had been studying finance at university and during the semester break he went travelling through South-East Asia, a trip documented by photographs on the wall by his hospital bed. Exactly what a 21-year-old should be doing. On his return, something changed. He was tired all the time and staying awake during classes became a mammoth effort. A cold or flu, he thought, and shrugged it off. Week by week and then day by day, he felt his body betraying him. Fluid filled his legs, his lungs and his belly. He could barely move from his bed and finally gave in to his mother's pleas to see a doctor.

Michael assumed it was probably some tropical illness picked up on his holiday of a lifetime; it couldn't have been further from his mind that his heart was failing. Badly. Michael's local doctor sent him in an ambulance to our hospital where he was admitted to the intensive care unit, poked and prodded and fitted with tubes and monitors that tracked all of his vital signs. Medicines were delivered by huge drips in his neck, to aid his heart to pump and reduce the fluid on his lungs. A small pump was placed next to his heart via the arteries in his groin. Despite the best medicines, Michael was getting sicker. Which is why I was standing at the end of his bed, looking at a grey man.

Michael's heart had been severely damaged. We will probably never know by what, maybe a virus, or a tiny segment of a gene. Either way, it was failing to a point where it couldn't support the rest of his body; his kidneys were already starting to fail from a lack of blood supply. Michael had a choice: take his chances and wait for a donor heart to become available, or undergo surgery to put in place two mechanical pumps, one for each side of his heart, then get strong enough to have a heart transplant.

In reality, he was too sick to wait for a donor heart. Getting greyer and greyer by the hour, Michael ended up with just one choice and that was to have two pumps fitted to keep him alive. In an operation that took five hours and tested his body more than ever before, Michael's ailing heart was helped by two ventricular assist devices (VADs) small enough to fit into the palm of a hand. Shiny metal was plugged into each side of his heart, carrying blood from the pump to the aorta and pulmonary artery.

Michael recovered and then he waited. The periods of waiting were interspersed with periods of problems, some big, some small. Regardless, when a donor heart became available, all of those months of waiting for Michael were in some ways over. In other ways, his journey was just beginning. Recovering from a huge surgery, his story switched from his broken heart to caring for this beautiful gift.

Transplantation was, and still is, seen as the pinnacle of what medicine can do for sick hearts, putting our knowledge and skill to the test like nothing else. The fact that we can take a heart from one person and give it to another, then have it beat, is amazing. It never stops being amazing to most of us involved in transplants. I know for a fact that for those lucky enough to receive this second chance, they too are amazed and exceptionally grateful.

As for Michael, I haven't seen him for a number of years but I hear he's living the full and wonderful life that a young man deserves, and that is the best gift anyone could ask for.

What is heart failure?

The vast majority of people who need a heart transplant (or VAD) have heart failure. Heart failure is the blanket term for a number of conditions that occur because the activity of the heart is no longer good enough to keep up with the demands of blood supply for the body.

There are an estimated 23 million people around the world living with heart failure. That number grew threefold from 1989 to 1999 and continues to climb. Scientific predictions are that one in every five people is at risk for heart failure in their lifetime. That's a huge number. And people with heart failure survive on average around 2.5 years from the time of diagnosis; a little less for women.

Heart failure can be an incredibly debilitating disease. Michael, who was bedbound and hooked up to machines and medicines, represents one extreme. There are many more people who are living at home with symptoms of heart failure that make their day-to-day lives tough. Their ankles swell to several times their normal size because the body hangs on to extra fluid due to hormones. These hormones, such as aldosterone, are desperately trying to correct the low output of the heart by giving the heart more fluid to pump.

The heart beats faster too, in an effort to try and make up for its poor pumping. A sick heart that beats too fast uses more oxygen and energy, energy that it can't necessarily get. Blood backs up around the body, including in the abdomen, so sufferers lose their appetite and sometimes an enormous amount of weight, a condition called cachexia where the body consumes all energy stores (fat and muscle) to stay alive.

The sicker people move from bed to chair and bathroom and back again. They need help with a lot of things that most of us do ourselves. Even mild forms of heart failure can dictate what you do in your life, and what you can't do.

Heart failure isn't just one problem, it is the end product of a number of conditions. Repeated heart attacks from blockages of the coronary arteries is known as **ischaemic cardiomyopathy**. Ischaemic means that there is insufficient blood supply and cardiomyopathy quite literally means 'heart muscle disease'. The heart is scarred and inefficient. As heart attacks and coronary artery disease becomes more common, the reality is that more and more people in the population are at risk for this type of heart failure.

The other types of heart failure include **dilated cardiomy-opathy**, which is when the heart dilates due to a disease of the heart muscle. Sometimes this follows an infection, such as a virus, that attacks the heart. Sometimes it happens in families because of genes that produce abnormal building blocks of the heart muscle cells. A type of heart failure that is commonly found in families is **hypertrophic cardiomyopathy**, when the heart muscle grows to a point where it can't work anymore and even stops blood flowing out of the heart. Hypertrophic refers to the process of hypertrophy, when muscle cells grow abnormally thick.

Heart valves, which keep blood moving in the correct directions, can fail, becoming too tight (**stenotic**) or very leaky (**regurgitant**), meaning the heart has to work harder than it should. **Valvular heart disease** is a common cause of heart failure in the developing world, where illnesses such as rheumatic fever are still quite common. Even in a developed country, Aboriginal Australians are still getting rheumatic fever and it's a common reason for them to develop heart failure, even in young people.

Sometimes we don't know why someone's heart decided to fail; we refer to the condition as 'idiopathic', which essentially translates as 'unknown'. I know our disappointment as healthcare workers when we have no explanation, but receiving the diagnosis of a serious illness without knowing the cause must be extraordinarily difficult to take.

Over the years, doctors and researchers have developed medicines to help patients with heart failure feel better, and to help them live longer. One of the first treatments we use is **diuretics** – medicines that help the body pee out more fluid. Since a lot of symptoms come from having too much fluid on the lungs or in the limbs and abdomen, losing this extra fluid can give quite a bit of relief.

The rest of the medicines we use are essentially aimed at reducing stress on the heart, much of which has happened because of the body's sometimes overzealous compensation. We use drugs called **beta-blockers** that slow the heart rate and stop it essentially being flogged while it's sick, and angiotensin converting enzyme inhibitors, or **ACE inhibitors** for short, that reduce the stress on the heart from blood pressure and may also help the heart heal a little if it has the ability to.

A lot of people are living day to day on these medicines. But not everyone is that well. When a heart is so broken that even medicines don't help it, the only way forward is to get a shiny new heart.

Metal hearts

Former US vice-president Dick Cheney started smoking cigarettes at the age of 12, helping them down with a packet of doughnuts. When he was running for Congress at the young age of 37, he had his first heart attack, one of five he would have over his lifetime. By 2010 Cheney was a cardiac cripple, suffering with end-stage heart failure. He found a new lease of life when he was fitted with a metal 'mechanical heart'.

Just like Michael, Cheney stayed attached to his pump until a donor heart became available. In years gone by, it's possible neither Cheney nor Michael nor some of the thousands of people who have had this incredible technology fitted would have survived. It changed the way we treat heart failure. Colloquially referred to as a mechanical heart, the VAD takes over some, often most, of the work of the ailing heart.

The 1960s were big for heart surgery and it was in 1966 that Dr Michael DeBakey implanted the first successful LVAD (left ventricular assist device) into a patient. The device stayed there for 10 days and the patient, who had undergone open-heart surgery, recovered. It was a bumpy road ahead for VADs but they remained the holy grail for treating heart failure. In 1967 the first heart transplant took place in South Africa; however, heart transplants were not as reliable then as they are today, and many patients died in the days and weeks after the procedure.

It wasn't until the mid-2000s that a large trial showed that patients who had an LVAD (pronounced *el-vad*) survived longer with heart failure than people that were only given the best medicines available. After that, VADs really took off. All of the major regulatory bodies around the world, such as the Food and Drug Administration (FDA) in the United States, approved these new-generation devices for use in patients who were awaiting a heart transplant.

Even during my career VADs have changed the face of heart failure. Take Michael, for example. He was able to go home, get strong and be in the best possible condition when a heart transplant eventually became possible. Now, around the world, approximately half of all patients have some form of machine in place when they get a transplant.

When I first started in cardiac surgery, VADs were huge, clunky devices. Around 2005, the first LVAD patient I saw receiving a heart transplant had an LVAD that weighed 1150 grams. Early VADs were connected to huge consoles, like shopping trolleys, that meant although patients' ailing hearts were taken care of, the patients were confined to their rooms and absolutely confined to hospital. Some devices weren't as durable as they are now and we really had to hope for a donor heart to come along quickly.

Previously, patients were on these devices for a little under a year on average. Now, at my hospital, we have a patient who has had an LVAD for 10 years and has travelled the world. The current generation of devices are smaller and more reliable than ever before. One of the smallest approved devices available now weighs only 160 grams. They've been trimmed down to the point that they fit inside your hand.

The technology behind VADs is pretty cool. They work by providing a continuous flow of blood from the heart, through the pump and out around the body. The pump is plugged into the left ventricle for an LVAD (or the right for an RVAD – right ventricular assist device) and sucks blood from the heart into the pump housing.

There are two main types of devices currently in widespread use and each works a little differently. One is a centrifugal pump: its motor spins and blood is spun to the outside of the shell before whooshing forward. It's the same kind of principle as the rides at the fairground where you defy gravity. The other one uses an axial flow: blood is pushed in the same direction as the motor. Either way, both pumps work quite differently to the heart. Both types are driven by magnets: when an electrical current is applied through them, they cause the pump to spin and displace blood.

Normally, the heart beats and squeezes in a rhythmical, intermittent manner. It's what gives you a pulse. If you feel your own pulse, that push against your fingers is the heart pushing blood out through your circulatory system. People who have an LVAD have no pulse. None at all. There's no intermittent push of blood, just continuous, nonstop blood flow. A patient of ours who has an LVAD loves being the guinea pig for first-aid training, purely to watch the look on people's faces when they can't find the pulse.

From that shiny metal pump, the blood is forced out through a piece of tubing that connects the pump to the aorta, if it's an LVAD, or the pulmonary artery, if it's an RVAD. Most adults pump around four to five litres of blood a minute around the body and the VAD can do pretty similar numbers. One thing that we can't yet achieve is to get the VAD to know when we're exercising and turn up the flow. It's an important area of interest, especially if we want these pumps to be used more widely.

The power for the VAD is something else that researchers are working on because, at the moment, they have to be plugged in. Not to a socket like some kind of cyborg, but their owner wears a battery pack in a bag that connects to a drive line. The drive line pierces the abdomen and connects to the VAD giving it power and telling it what to do, how fast to turn the pump and getting information back, such as how much power it's using.

Most of us put in VADs using a form of open-heart surgery. It's a really wonderful operation because usually when the patient comes into the operating theatre, they look sick. Some are dying before our eyes; others are maxed out on the best possible medications that we can give them. When the chest is opened, the pump is sewn to the heart. As it takes over, the heart almost visibly sighs, like it's finally getting a reprieve from its struggle. The patient leaves the operating theatre often looking better than when they came in, which is why it's such a satisfying and rewarding thing to be a part of.

People with VADs can do nearly anything. Every year, a group of our VAD patients participate in a fun run called the City to Surf. They usually walk the four-kilometre race and I can promise you, they do not bring up the rear. They go back to work, drive cars and go on holidays. It's a far cry from the days when people with such severe heart failure would be essentially bedbound.

Most people who have a VAD are what we call 'bridge to transplant', in that the VAD is keeping them alive and well until a donor heart becomes available. A smaller proportion are grouped into 'destination therapy', which means they have their VAD until the day that they die. Which, coincidentally, is the day their VAD is turned off. These patients for whatever reason don't tick all the boxes necessary for a heart transplant.

The future may bring VADs that are even safer, more durable and more sophisticated than those we have now. It may be a possibility that heart transplants are taken over by these shiny, new, metal hearts. Researchers and clinicians everywhere are working on making VADs even better so that perhaps one day, people won't have to sit waiting for the precious gift of a donor heart to be given.

How to perform a heart transplant

A heart transplant goes a little something like this. A patient, who is waiting for a heart, gets a call. It's the call they have often been waiting to get for months or even longer. They're told, 'We have a suitable donor heart for you and you need to get into the hospital'.

At the same time, someone has died and their family has made the incredibly difficult yet courageous choice to donate their organs, to give someone else a chance. They have generally had some kind of catastrophic brain injury from an accident or a burst blood vessel, for example. They are what we call brain dead, meaning that their brain is no longer working and can't send vital messages to the rest of the body. It's completely unrecoverable.

A team of doctors from the transplant hospital travel to that donor and perform an operation to retrieve the heart or other organs. It's a special operation and a sombre one. There are very few times when you walk into an operating theatre and find that respect is quite that palpable. In these rooms, we're fully mindful of the very special significance of what we're about to do, receiving the gift of an organ for someone who desperately needs it.

I remember one retrieval, from a young man who had died after an accident. His mother could not come to see her son, yet made that incredible decision to donate his heart. As is routine before any surgery, we check all the paperwork including the consent for surgery. From afar, his mother had given consent over the phone and we listened to a phone recording of that conversation. Not the first time this had happened, but it may have been the first time there wasn't a dry eye in the operating theatre.

The donor heart is stopped with a special preservation solution that keeps the heart cold and safe while it's transported back to the home hospital. For the time being at least, keeping the heart cold in a cool-box filled with ice is how we look after the heart. A cold heart has virtually no requirement for oxygen or other energy, as long as we can get it into our recipient within around four to six hours. It means it's often a mad dash back to the hospital, sometimes in police cars or jets. Sometimes both.

The recipient will be asleep; once the all clear is given by the donor team, the implant team start the operation to remove their heart. They're supported on a heart–lung machine, also called a **cardiopulmonary bypass machine**, which does the work of the heart and lungs. The patient is connected to it by a series of tubes, and a clamp across the aorta isolates the heart from the rest of the body.

It's an eerie experience to look into someone's chest and see it empty. Once the old sick heart is out of the body, the implant of the healthy new one starts. It feels like kilometres of sewing: the left atrium, the pulmonary artery, the aorta, the superior and inferior vena cava. 'Time is heart' and once it's time to put the new one in, we sew quickly and methodically.

That's not the best part. The best part is when we remove a clamp and blood is allowed to come rushing back to the new heart. One of my favourite things about the heart is this: when you give the heart (or even heart cells) nutrient-rich, oxygenated blood, it just starts beating. And this is, by and large, what the new heart does. It's sometimes like a little deer at first, trying to find its legs walking for the first time. And then it learns what to do, and it just beats.

I often feel at the point when the heart begins to take over and work well that there is a collective sigh of relief in the room. Like we've all been waiting to make sure it works and everything is fine. Once inside its new chest, the heart is awfully clever, and it has to be. The heart is normally connected to our brains and nervous systems by nerves that send messages to the heart, especially to the pacemaker centres of the heart, the **sinoatrial node**, which is responsible for keeping the beat, so to speak. Since the new heart doesn't get these signals anymore to speed up or slow down, it has to work it out another way. The nerves to the heart are cut and can't really be rejoined at the time of the transplant. Which brings me to the next thing I love about the heart.

The heart will handle any blood that you give it. It just pumps out what it gets. When we exercise, we increase the blood returning to the heart as the working muscles squeeze it back into our chests. The heart realises that it has more blood and so it has a kind of reflex and starts pumping harder and faster. Some heart transplant recipients say that they can feel that lag while the heart realises it's time to work, but after that, well, they can carry on as they need.

The transplanted heart beats a little faster than a native heart, maybe up to ninety times a minute compared with sixty to seventy for the rest of us. The lack of connection to a nerve supply to the parasympathetic nervous system, and specifically the vagal nerve branches, means that the new heart doesn't get the 'calm down' signals at rest that regular hearts do. Not having the nerves connected also means that at maximal effort, a heart transplant patient may not be able to keep up with someone who hasn't had one. I say 'may not' because there are transplanted athletes who are fitter than most of us who haven't had a heart transplant!

Heart transplantation is not so much a cure for heart failure, but a treatment. We are literally cutting out the old sick heart to replace it with a new one. Life after a heart transplant can be incredibly rich. A number of recipients participate in sport; some even do gruelling triathlons. However, it does come with a set of responsibilities, needs and longer-term worries.

The main thing we worry about after heart transplant is rejection. Our bodies' immune systems are very carefully trained to recognise when something does not belong, whether that be an infection or the tissue or organs from another person (or animal). The immune system attacks anything that it doesn't recognise as its own. To stop the new heart being attacked, transplant patients are on a cocktail of medications called **immunosuppressants** that dull the immune system so the heart isn't attacked.

The downside of immunosuppression is that the transplant recipient is left open to infection. They often take long-term antibiotics to ward off hard-to-treat infections. While they seem like a burden, these drugs are life-saving. In the early days of transplants, the only medications we had to stop rejection were steroids. They bombed out the immune system so much that most recipients died within days or weeks, from overwhelming infection. The discovery of cyclosporine in the early 1980s allowed transplant to forge ahead without devastating infections lurking.

Over time, a transplanted heart can develop problems, especially if there have been periods of rejection. It is possible to receive a second heart transplant. Australian Fiona Coote received two heart transplants as a child in Sydney after her first one failed. She has lived nearly 32 years after her second transplant. Over time, however, the heart can begin to fail or develop thickening of the coronary arteries. Which is why it's not so much of a cure but a very high-level treatment for heart failure.

Today, after a heart transplant, people live on average for around 12 years – although a lot live longer. That time has improved progressively as we get better at looking after patients who have had transplants. That includes new drugs, better care of the donor heart and simply more experience with these patients. Today, 85 per cent of people survive the first year and this group in particular do very well in the long term. John McCafferty received a heart transplant in London in 1982 and survived 33 years, dying at 71. He was one of the longest-surviving recipients of a heart transplant.

Cravings and new loves

A common dinner-party question: do heart transplant recipients take on the characteristics of their donors? It's a decent question considering, every now and again, we will read about someone who woke up from a transplant and craved a beer although they used to hate it. Some decide to take up a sport or a hobby that they hadn't done before. Some people have even claimed to have dreamt of their donor.

So what's the science? People do sometimes change after their transplant. A study in Austria found that 79 per cent of people who received a heart transplant felt they had no change in their personality at all. The rest thought that they had changed, but only a small minority thought it was because of their new heart. Most thought that it was because of the life-threatening illness changing their outlook on life.

Even though we know better now, the heart still represents our emotional core in a cultural sense. Some people imagine they would have trouble accepting the idea of having another's heart, or perhaps giving their heart away because it is their soul, their essence. It possibly explains why we want to believe in personality changes after a transplant. There's not much science to support the idea that a heart transplant recipient may take up a new hobby because the new heart suggests it, but having a 'change of heart' regarding life after a major illness? Well, that makes perfect sense.

Organ donation

It's hard to talk about heart transplant without talking about how those hearts come to be. A donated heart comes from somebody who has died; as we have already mentioned, usually from a catastrophic brain injury, when a person has been declared brain dead. Brain death occurs when there is irreversible loss of function of the brain; it can't be recovered from. To be certain that a patient is brain dead, two doctors do a battery of tests independently to ensure that the patient has indeed passed away. It's an incredibly ethical and strict process to protect the patient. At this point, organ donation has nothing to do with the process.

In Australia around 69 per cent of people are willing to be organ donors, but only around 1 or 2 per cent die in the very special set of circumstances required to be an organ donor. They have to be in an intensive care unit and closely monitored. The situation is similar in the United Kingdom and United States, with the final decision being left up to the family. The United States has one of the better donor rates around the world, while Australia is ranked twentieth. All of this means that we have a desperate shortage of organs for people who are waiting for their chance to have a transplant.

Many of us don't talk about whether or not we would like to be an organ donor if we die. That means in most countries, that decision falls to our grieving families. In some countries like Spain and Belgium, an opt-out system exists where everyone is considered to be a donor unless they specifically register their wishes not to be.

I don't often get to see the other side. Rules strictly prohibit the transplant teams having anything to do with the care of the donor, to keep everything strictly ethical. However, I have over the years been privy to two separate cases of families who have donated organs and count it as a bright light to come out of a very dark situation.

One was a colleague of mine whose mother passed away after a road accident. The family made the decision to donate her organs. It was a hard time for the family to lose their mother: there were babies on the way and weddings in the future. However, they remain steadfast in believing that donation was the right decision; they healed so much knowing that someone would have a second chance at life as a result of their mother's gift.

The other was a recipient who, through a series of very strange coincidences, ran into her donor family. They struck up a relationship that persists to this day. Every time they're together, their loved one is with them, beating away inside another's chest. The heart lives on, as does the reminder of the beautiful gift that they all chose to share.

Preventing heart failure

Heart failure is growing to be one of the biggest threats to health of our time. Unless you're among the group who suffer an unfortunate infection, an unknown cause or a genetic predisposition to have heart failure, it's largely preventable. Nearly a third of transplants worldwide are performed because of coronary artery disease damaging the heart, usually over many years. Other diseases, such as valve disease, that lead to heart failure can often be treated early before the heart muscle is irrevocably damaged.

To reduce your lifetime risk of heart failure, reducing your risk of coronary disease is pivotal. Eat a balanced diet and exercise regularly, as exercise is a great way of preventing heart disease. If you smoke, it's time to quit right away; the sooner you do, the sooner your body can start healing. In men who were thought to be at risk of heart failure, studies show that taking up at least four healthy lifestyle factors (exercise, diet, weight loss, not smoking) reduced their risk of heart failure from 21 per cent to 10 per cent.

Most importantly, know your heart. Just as for heart disease, make sure that you know your risk factors. Know your blood pressure and your cholesterol and be checked for diabetes. Have your heart checked if you are at risk.

Although there's no doubt that there have been wonderful modern developments in heart transplants and mechanical hearts, the best attitude to adopt is that you have only one heart. Take care of it as if it was as beautiful a gift as a donated heart.

chapter 4
THE MEDICAL MYSTERIES OF A WOMAN'S HEART

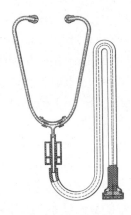

A woman's heart is a deep ocean of secrets
ROSE, *TITANIC*

If I told you a woman's heart is different to a man's, would you think I was stating the obvious? Of course I am, but not for the reasons you might think. Did you know that heart disease is *the* leading cause of death in women? This is one of the biggest untold stories of women's health, under-acknowledged by women and healthcare professionals alike. Women's hearts are structurally different to men's and they experience heart attacks differently, but most of the research done into heart attacks has been done by men, on men. When a woman has a heart attack, she is more likely to die than a man. And younger women are especially at risk. That is all changing though, as we learn more about what makes a woman's heart tick.

Our society has traditionally portrayed a woman's heart in books, films and fairytales as something fragile and delicate, a prize to be won or broken by someone who doesn't reciprocate her love. That's not strictly true, of course. A woman's heart is much more than romantic fodder. And it can be both life-giving and life-threatening.

I once had a patient whose story really got to me. She was not much older than me and when we first met she was on life support in the intensive care unit. Despite that, I felt like I knew her because the walls of the ICU room were covered in photographs of her smiling at the camera, fit and healthy. She could have been me.

A few days earlier, she had been getting ready for a lunch party for her father. She didn't make it to the party because while she was getting ready, she suddenly felt incredibly ill. Her breathing became laboured and she had chest pains. Sweat poured down her face and she stumbled backwards, calling for her husband and her children to help. They drove her to the local emergency department, luckily not even five minutes away. I say luckily because as they arrived, her heart stopped beating. As the doctors and nurses started pushing on her chest and giving her medicines, her heart sprang back into action. She had suffered a heart attack. But why? Young, fit and healthy: logic would tell us it shouldn't happen to her.

A test was done, called a **coronary angiogram**. A special kind of dye is injected into the coronary arteries to check if they are blocked. In this case, the main artery of the heart had torn, causing a massive heart attack. This is called a **spontaneous coronary artery dissection** and is almost exclusively seen in women under the age of 50 or in women who have recently given birth. This wasn't a small dissection either. The heart muscle and the whole of her left ventricle had been so badly damaged that it didn't pump anymore, it barely quivered. Suddenly, the smiling woman in the photos, swimming and hugging friends, was dependent on the most advanced machines and medicines to keep her alive.

A few days after this, she came to the operating theatre for another life-saving procedure. She underwent the insertion of an LVAD mechanical heart. This pump will keep her alive while she waits for a transplant, when her sick heart and the pump will be removed and replaced with a healthy donor heart.

I saw in this woman someone not too dissimilar to myself. Yet she had been struck down. It has resonated with me for years as I watched women with heart problems come through the hospital. Some have hearts that were not formed properly before their birth, and some are burdened by diabetes, high blood pressure or bad genes. Some are just plain unlucky.

Oestrogen and blood vessels

Even up until the late 1990s heart disease wasn't seen as something that generally affected women. In fact, an important medical journal once published an article declaring that, because the risk of heart attack to women was much lower than men, they didn't need to worry about it. And neither did their doctors.

This myth sprang from two things: a bit of hormones and a bit of maths. Up until menopause, women make oestrogen. Oestrogen is a pretty great hormone to have around because it protects against some diseases. Oestrogen helps keep your bones strong so you don't get osteoporosis (when bones weaken and thin and break more easily). In the heart and blood vessels, oestrogen acts as an almost perfect antidote to heart disease. For a hormone that is made by, and mostly for, a woman's reproductive organs, it does a kick-ass job elsewhere.

You remember cholesterol and bad fats? These little beasts almost burrow into the walls of the blood vessels, bringing with them all kinds of cells, including **macrophages**. Macrophages are an important part of your immune system: fighting infection, inflammation and even cancer. They are, however, a bit aggressive when they turn up in the wall of the blood vessel and they attack the cholesterol. The macrophage bites off more than it can chew, swelling full of fat and turning into a foam cell. The attack and the response cause a swelling in the wall of the blood vessel, making a plaque, which, as it grows, obstructs blood flow down that vessel, causing a stroke or heart attack.

Oestrogen is very good at calming down this process in many ways. When the fats are trying to invade and the macrophages are inadvertently injuring the vessel, oestrogen comes along and sends the fats, macrophages and any of their plaque-causing buddies on their way, leaving the blood vessels relatively plaque free. The oestrogen sends signals to calm down inflammation in the walls of blood vessels and sends cholesterol to be stored where it can't damage blood vessels. It also helps blood vessels relax and stay supple so that they can stretch to get bigger and keep blood flowing. Oestrogens are the blood vessels' yoga teachers, relaxing them and cleansing everyone.

Doctors and scientists started to think that oestrogen had an important role to play in heart disease for two reasons. Firstly, after menopause women start to have a lot more heart attacks and, when we look at the coronary arteries, a lot more blockages. In fact, they get more blockages in all of the arteries of the body after menopause. The second red flag was that women who were taking synthetic oestrogens in hormone replacement therapy (HRT) seemed to be having fewer heart attacks and fewer blockages of their arteries than women who weren't on HRT. You're probably thinking 'oestrogen prevents heart disease, so why don't we all just take oestrogen?' and, really, that's a great question. After all, we give HRT to women to alleviate the symptoms of menopause, such as brittle bones or hot flushes. There are two main reasons why we don't prescribe HRT for the heart alone: studies showed that HRT didn't do as good a job as we had hoped when given to women to prevent arteries from developing blockages; and for some women HRT might increase the risk of breast cancer or clots in the legs and lungs (deep vein thrombosis). Essentially, the risks are not worth the benefits when it comes to looking after your heart. This is a great conversation to have with your doctor to see what the benefits would be for you.

Precisely how oestrogen and other hormones and biological differences between men and women affect the heart and its health is currently under intense investigation. We have enough evidence to tell us that the link is definitely there, but the nitty-gritty of the mechanism is something we're still learning about. When we learn more about that mechanism, we might even be able to develop it into a treatment.

A feminine heart

Looking specifically at women's hearts and heart disease is relatively new and it is showing some fascinating and very important findings. This research has shown how women develop disease differently to men and respond differently if they do. And this isn't just interesting and unusual scientific note-taking: it's vitally important that we work this out, because heart disease is killing women.

For years, research into heart disease has been very male focused. There are a few reasons for this and a lot of it is to do with how research is conducted. For a research trial, people with a disease, such as heart disease, are enlisted and given a medication or a procedure, then we see how they go. We watch if the disease gets better or if patients feel better or even if there are more deaths than in another group who are having a different treatment. Since men have more heart attacks, over the years more men were recruited to these trials. So we've based our tests and our treatments on results from men.

However, while it's true that men have more heart attacks than women, when women have heart attacks they don't fare as well as the guys. Women who have heart attacks die at higher rates than men, and the survivors have more heart failure, which makes doing normal things really tough. In younger women, this difference is particularly bad. If you're a woman under 50 years of age and you have a heart attack, then you are twice as likely to die than a man in the same boat. Call me crazy, but that is just too big a difference to tolerate. When I read statistics like that, my first question is 'why?' and my second is 'what can we do about it?', but we will get to that later.

Here's the deal with women's hearts: they are biologically different. Very different, in fact. Let's start with the simple things... a woman's heart is smaller than a man's. That doesn't make it an inferior model; it still gets the job done. It usually beats a little faster than a man's, although, depending on your level of fitness, even that difference might not exist. These are not the important differences though; it is the inner workings that really matter. The first difference is very interesting. A heart attack happens when the arteries that supply blood to the heart are blocked by plaque made from fats and cells of the immune system. That's the conventional heart attack and, if we do a coronary angiogram, as the dye flows down the arteries we can actually see it stop at a blockage in the artery. Except when it doesn't. There is another way to have a heart attack and it often happens to women.

Imagine you're stuck in traffic. You're caught on the motorway because a mile up ahead there is a truck broken down in the left lane. Everyone has to try and squeeze around that truck and it makes the remaining road really narrow. That's the first type of heart attack: a big blockage smack bang in the way. Now imagine that road workers have placed bright orange cones along the road, on both sides, making the whole stretch of road narrow. You don't have to squeeze past one discrete area of a breakdown, but squeezing through a narrower road slows you down. That's similar to how heart attacks can happen in women.

The way women develop plaque in the coronary arteries is a lot more like narrowing the whole section of road on both sides. This has a couple of side effects that mean women can get a raw deal when it comes to winning the war against heart disease. The first is that it's hard to see on tests such as coronary angiograms. Just like looking down on the traffic jam, there's no discrete blockage on the angiogram. Angiograms are great for spotting bigger blockages, but not as good at seeing the orange cones.

The second side effect is how the female arteries behave and respond. Coronary arteries have muscle in their wall and this can contract, narrowing the vessel, or relax, making it wide open. Female arteries are much more likely to contract really hard, causing narrowing and a traffic jam for the blood.

Blood vessels are lined with a bunch of clever cells, making up a lining called the **endothelium** (*en-DOH-thee-lee-um*). Not content with just watching blood go by, the endothelium has lots of important roles. It releases hormones that can make blood vessels relax or contract and it sends out signals when it's damaged to create blood clots so we don't bleed all over the place. When it's misbehaving, it can create all kinds of havoc, such as muscle contraction to make the artery tiny, or promoting the production of plaque that causes blockages over time. Factors such as too many bad fats, smoking and high blood pressure can send the clever endothelium crazy, so it goes rogue.

The heart muscle is also a little different in women. When the heart muscle contracts, we call this **systole** (*sis-tol-ee*). Usually when someone develops heart failure, it refers to the fact that the pumping action of the heart is not great. If the heart can't pump well, the organs and tissues of the body don't get the blood, oxygen and nutrients that they need. But there is another cause of heart failure. When the heart muscle relaxes we call this period of time **diastole** (*dye-as-tol-ee*). Diastole is a very important time for the heart – it is when all the blood comes rushing back into the heart, ready to be pushed out around the body.

Let's imagine for a second that the heart is a balloon. When it's empty, it is soft. As you add air, or perhaps water, the walls of the balloon stretch. Then they aren't so soft and squishy: the balloon is much firmer and its surface feels tense and looks shiny. Now let's imagine a balloon with a really thick, stiff wall. That's going to be much harder to fill. The wall is too stiff to expand as you blow air into it, and the heart can be the same. The medical term is **diastolic dysfunction** – a heart that is far too stiff to fill effectively. This means the heart simply can't get enough blood inside to have a decent volume to shoot around the body. That is an incredible thing about the heart: with every beat it ejects the blood it receives. If it doesn't have enough blood inside, then it struggles to pump that small volume effectively around the body. This stiff heart is very hard to treat, people who have it feel quite unwell and the rates of death are higher than in other types of heart failure. Unfortunately, it's also more common in women.

Are you starting to feel that women have been dealt a bad hand in the heart disease stakes? There's still more, because we're yet to consider one of the biggest differences between men's and women's bodies.

Baby-making

Babies are the big difference between men and women. And if you ask a woman who has had children for a list of symptoms that occurred when she was pregnant, she'll probably tell you about swollen ankles, constipation or reflux. Despite the wonderful reward at the end, most women would agree that being pregnant is a big stress on their bodies.

They're right. Those nine months place a huge amount of stress on the body and particularly on the heart. To look after the baby a woman's body is carrying, the heart beats faster and pushes more blood around the body to get nutrients to the baby. That's not all though. A woman's blood vessels become softer and stretch due to pregnancy hormones, and other processes occur that we're not even sure about yet.

Pregnancy can be such a big stress on the body that it can create disease that especially impacts on the heart. Certain diseases can show themselves in pregnancy and what we're now sure of is that the women who develop these problems have to be extra careful for the rest of their lives.

The first issue that can affect a woman's heart during and after pregnancy is **gestational diabetes**. Diabetes that occurs during pregnancy is a big problem for both mother and baby. It can make the baby grow very large, making the birth risky for baby and mother, and can make the baby really sick after birth. Babies born to diabetic mums are also more likely to develop diabetes themselves later in life. It also means that the mother is at risk of other serious pregnancy complications.

The other serious disease in pregnancy is **pre-eclampsia**. This occurs when the mother's blood pressure gets very high and her kidneys leak a lot of protein. Left untreated it leads to **eclampsia,** when the kidneys, liver and blood cells are affected. The worst cases lead to seizures. Just as with diabetes, a sick mum means a sick baby. Some women get high blood pressure in pregnancy and, while it's not as severe as having pre-eclampsia or eclampsia, it is something important to be aware of.

Both of these problems usually improve after the baby has been delivered. Even though things 'settle down' and return to normal, problems with blood pressure or diabetes in pregnancy unmask a woman who is prone to these conditions. Diabetes and high blood pressure are some of the most common risks for heart disease. They are responsible for directly harming the body's blood vessels and heart. They may disappear after childbirth, but their after-effects are felt for years to come. Doctors and nurses are becoming much more aware that women who have had diabetes or pre-eclampsia during pregnancy need to be watched much more closely than those that didn't. These women need to be extra cautious to take good care of themselves for years to come.

Problems that plague women's hearts

* Pregnancy can be a 'stress test', causing direct harm to the heart and unmasking women who are at risk in the future.
* Polycystic ovary syndrome can make women more likely to be overweight, which is not helpful in keeping your heart healthy.
* Women are susceptible to problems with their immune system, such as overactivity. These autoimmune diseases can place extra stress on the heart or can make the heart sick.
* Some diseases of the heart are more common in women, such as spontaneous coronary artery dissection, diastolic heart failure or peripartum cardiomyopathy (when the heart pumps very poorly after giving birth).
* Diseases like diabetes are much more harmful to a woman's heart than a man's. Women who have diabetes get more frequent and more severe complications of the disease.

Heart attacks aren't like they are in the movies

Movies and TV have taught us quite a bit about heart attacks. They tend to usually go the same way: someone, almost always a man, clutches their chest and appears to be in absolute agony. They fall to the ground and roll around and are then surrounded by onlookers, before someone rushes in and announces they are a doctor. If the heart stops, someone gives **CPR** and the patient makes a miraculous recovery. Jack Nicholson recovers from a heart attack to annoy Diane Keaton in *Something's Gotta Give*, his backside hanging out of his hospital gown, and all ends well.

Whether you're male or female, that is not usually how things go. Most people report chest pain as the predominant symptom of a heart attack, but it's not often that dramatic. It's most commonly called 'crushing', like 'having an elephant on your chest' was how one man described it to me many years ago. Sometimes, the pain travels up your jaw or down your arms or even through your back. Many patients report feeling very sick and some vomit. Others get sweaty and pale as their bodies make lots of adrenaline to address the sudden insult to the heart. Sometimes this goes away if they sit down and rest. Sometimes it doesn't. Hollywood would be bored out of its mind with what a real heart attack looks like.

Women are a little more subtle when they have heart attacks. That classic crushing chest pain is less common in women. Only around half of women who have a heart attack report this as a symptom. Women have other tricky symptoms which are hard for doctors or nurses to pick up on, and make it hard for women themselves to work out if something really is wrong. Women have pain in funny places such as the jaw or the top of the belly, or sometimes just the back. They may get incredibly tired or short of breath doing things they used to be able to do, like taking the stairs or walking the dog.

Whenever I say this, every woman in the room rolls her eyes at me and says, 'Well I'm always tired, surely that's not my heart!' and happily they're right. It illustrates a vital point though. It's tough to tease out what is just life or simple back pain, and what is the serious stuff. That confusion is not just for the tired among us. Even doctors and nurses can be misled.

I got a phone call from a doctor who wanted me to do open-heart surgery on someone who had recently had a heart attack, and fix the blockages that had caused all the drama. He told me her story: she was in her late forties and a smoker; her dad had died of a heart attack at 50. He described how she came to the emergency department with what doctors call atypical chest pain. That means it's different from Hollywood-style chest pain; we often think it has nothing to do with the heart. Someone, though, had ordered blood tests that showed there was indeed a heart attack and when she had a test to look for blockages in the coronary arteries, they were there and they were bad.

I listened to the doctor and I heard wonderment in his voice. He seemed to be saying 'How weird is this? Isn't it just plain luck that someone checked?', as if we had stumbled upon the answer to a great mystery. This story is not unusual. So often, neither the patient nor the doctors put the pieces of the puzzle together and recognise that heart attacks can be tricksters. Heart attacks pretend to be something else or, even more commonly, they pretend to be nothing at all, like a room full of tired women.

I remember a colleague telling me about a young woman she had seen in her clinic. She was 40 years old and worked as a lawyer. She was fit and healthy, walking or running several times a week, had never smoked, hardly drank and looked after herself. Which may have been why nobody could work out why she couldn't walk as far as she used to. The reason she couldn't walk was that whenever she got a bit of speed on, she got this ache in the side of her neck. This woman had seen at least three doctors, all of whom scratched their heads and ordered blood tests and ultrasounds to look at her neck.

In a moment of desperation, she sought out this colleague of mine who just so happens to be a cardiologist and a woman. She's also a straight shooter. She told me she looked at this woman and said to her: 'I would be surprised if there was something wrong with your heart, you're so healthy and young. But, we should check.' So, they did. This fit, slim, healthy woman had a coronary angiogram to see if she had any blockages of her coronary arteries that were causing her neck pain. My colleague showed me the pictures and I gasped in horror as the film played on a screen. They had discovered the problem. This woman had a very tight, very unhealthy blockage in the biggest and possibly most important artery of the heart. This story has a happy ending: she had it treated and is well. But not everyone gets that sort of ending.

This woman with her neck pain and healthy lifestyle did not tick the boxes you need to tick to be given the right test, a coronary angiogram, until she saw someone who thought that something must be wrong. She just didn't fit the bill. Women are far less likely to be referred for these types of tests largely because they don't fit the bill of a 'typical' heart attack. Not only that, but, as we discovered earlier, it isn't always the right test.

Over time medicine has greatly improved how it treats heart disease. Unless you're a woman. You may be wondering why the ladies are once again coming off second best. To the best of my knowledge, there isn't a room full of faceless men deciding that the good pills are only going to the men. The truth is more complicated than that.

We already learnt that the way a woman's heart works is different to a man's, but the way it deals with disease is also different. When it comes to women's heart disease, we are dealing with a different beast.

Over the years, since medical trials were performed primarily on male volunteers, the concoction of medicines and surgery developed to battle heart disease have been tested on men. Who just so happen to have male-type heart disease. When we use the same armamentarium on women, the medicines and surgery haven't been refined for the kind of heart disease particular to women. They don't work as well and the combination that does hasn't been found yet.

When I consider all of these ways women fare so much worse than men when it comes to heart disease, I feel pretty annoyed, a bit sad and a little worried for my own heart health. It is a tricky situation – we can't do tests, especially invasive ones, on everyone with unusual symptoms, or simply based on suspicions and assumptions. Some tests carry risks and we try not to expose people to them unnecessarily. Researchers and doctors are currently looking at the tests we use on the heart, as well as new possibilities to work out how best to use them for women. Don't despair just yet: the tide is turning!

The future of women's hearts

Once an afterthought, women's heart disease is now getting a lot of attention. Around the world, researchers are probing into the questions of women's hearts and battling to unravel some of the mysteries. Research is being undertaken on the differences in biology of heart disease, to decipher how women's hearts behave, and hopefully lead to better treatments.

One of the most important things we can do is change the conversation, from heart disease being a man's disease to a woman's disease. Around the world, campaigns such as Go Red for Women and Making the Invisible Visible are geared towards raising awareness of heart disease for women, their families and healthcare workers.

Moving closer to home, what about the future of your own heart? Since women who develop heart disease don't do as well, prevention is much more important than cure. Much heart disease is preventable. Diabetes and high blood pressure are generally developed through years of habits, and 'lifestyle' factors also play a part. Added to this are our genes. Maybe we got lucky and have genes that protect us from heart disease; but then again, maybe we got ones that make life tougher.

A woman's heart is a beautiful thing, and that's not just in the movies or romance books. Think of all the women in your life, and how you want them all to live long and happy lives. While we work on unraveling the difficulties of the female heart, take care of your own with everything you have.

Caring for your heart: the woman's cheat sheet

Over 80 per cent of women have one preventable risk factor for heart disease, and 60 per cent have three or more. These are factors such as smoking, being overweight, physical inactivity, diabetes or high blood pressure. Talk to your doctor about how to get these under control.

* Know your risk factors. Talk to your family and see who has heart troubles, get your blood pressure and cholesterol checked and have a once-over for diabetes. Knowledge is power for change.
* If you had problems in pregnancy, make sure that you keep an even closer eye on your health, not just in subsequent pregnancies but all the time. Since you might have a slightly higher risk of developing problems such as diabetes or high blood pressure, take extra care of yourself and be sure your doctor does the same.

* *Move! If you walk briskly or run, even if you got the dud heart disease genes, you can reduce your risk of heart disease by up to half.*
* *Talk about it. While we build awareness, spread the word to everyone you know about women's hearts and empower everyone to look after themselves.*

chapter 5

CAN
LOVE
HEAL?

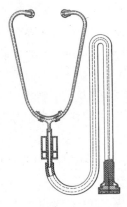

The best and most beautiful things in the world cannot be seen or even touched – they must be felt with the heart
HELEN KELLER, DEAF AND BLIND AUTHOR,
POLITICAL ACTIVIST AND LECTURER

When I was a junior doctor, doing my first rotation in cardiac surgery, seeing a heart beating in an open chest during my first heart surgery was awe-inspiring. But it wasn't the only aspect of the experience that inspired me. The patients did too – they were some of the bravest and most resilient people I had ever met.

One morning I came into work to find that we were performing a heart–lung transplant, a relatively rare surgery at that time. This was the transplant that would not only cement my decision to make a career in cardiac surgery, it was also one that would demonstrate to me the power of love.

Laura's story

Our patient was a wonderful woman called Laura. She had been born with a rare type of heart disease called **truncus arteriosus**. A normal heart has two large blood vessels leading out of it: the aorta and the pulmonary artery. Laura had only one main artery with one valve that didn't work very well. As a result, her heart and lungs were put under a lot of strain and her body received oxygen-poor blood, making her skin and lips blue. She was born at a time when heart surgery on babies wasn't advanced enough to fix the problem, so she had endured 40 years of illness and ever-worsening damage to her already sick heart and lungs.

The operation was a success. After nearly 10 hours of surgery, Laura was transferred to the intensive care unit where she was kept asleep to let her fragile new organs adapt to their new home. It was beautiful to see: her once dark-blue lips had turned a normal shade of pink as her new heart and lungs pumped blood in the right direction, filling her body with oxygen-rich blood.

Laura had been extremely sick before her surgery and her recovery was not smooth sailing. Along the way, there had been what I'd call collateral damage to a number of her other organs. When the body is already under stress, the organs can effectively revolt against the extra strain placed on them by surgery and recovery, not to mention the medicines required to keep everything working well. During the course of Laura's life, her body had confronted more stress than most. I remember during a ward round one evening, several weeks after Laura's surgery, I stood with other members of the medical team and lamented the fact that she had faced more obstacles than was reasonable for one person to shoulder.

I came to understand, however, that Laura wasn't shouldering this burden alone. I am sure that just as important as medicines or doctors in Laura's recovery was the support and constant presence of her husband, Andrew. He was loving her to better health. Slowly but surely, Laura overcame each challenge she faced during her recovery and was finally able to go home. Over the ensuing 10 years I have stayed in contact with Laura and Andrew and am constantly in awe of the way they have lived their lives together to the fullest.

The epicentre of love

In hospitals we see love all the time: it's the glue that binds people together. I often wonder how dependent a patient's recovery is on the love of another person. There is something about a patient being loved and loving back that pulls them towards recovery, towards health. Happily, most people don't need to experience something as traumatic as a heart–lung transplant to encounter love or its health benefits.

In the times of the ancient Greeks and Romans, philosophers and physicians from Aristotle to Galen viewed the heart as the focus of emotion, and the source of love, courage and compassion. People who were unkind were said to be 'dark-hearted' or 'black-hearted', implying that their actions were not only mean-spirited but also a dysfunction of their heart. Such terms suggested the dark heart lacked the goodness a heart should have. Love was the main feature of the heart's emotional repertoire, and terms of endearment such as 'sweetheart' are still used to refer to a person one loves.

Today we have a much greater understanding of the workings of the heart than those early philosophers. Despite this, and centuries of science showing us the true workings of our inner selves, we have never been able to let go of one idea: the heart remains strongly coupled to love. Matters relating to love are still called 'affairs of the heart'. In our cultures, our stories and our minds, the heart is viewed as the birthplace, epicentre and ruler of love.

The connection between the heart and love is not unfounded. Your heart beats faster when you see someone you love; it may even 'skip a beat'. But love is far more complex than simply being the response of a heartbeat. Feeling love or being loved by another person sets off a cascade of hormones and physical responses that don't just make you feel good, they're good for you, mind and body. In fact, even having self-compassion and love for yourself is healthy.

Hugs – how oxytocin is great for you

Think of the last time you were hugged. Not an awkward hug, but a hug from your significant other before you left for work, or from an old friend at the airport. The kind of hug that warms your soul and makes you feel loved. It's more than just the emotion of it – your body feels better after someone you love has hugged you.

No emotion is simply an emotion. We feel emotion in our physical being. Love is no exception. It has evolved into a biological and hormonal process inside us, centred around the hormone **oxytocin**. Oxytocin is often called the 'cuddle' or 'love' hormone but its role starts early in life, long before we know what love is. In a woman preparing to give birth, oxytocin is released by the pituitary gland, which sits nestled under the brain, causing her uterus to contract and push the baby out of the birth canal. It also causes milk to be expelled, enabling the baby to feed – one of the first true experiences of love we have.

A hormone is a molecule, usually a peptide (like a small protein), which is made in the cells of the body. Its job is to travel to other cells and cause changes in the way a cell functions. Hormones act as sophisticated little signalling molecules, kind of like a message that is passed around a room of people asking them to do (or not do) something. The organs and cells that make these hormones release them after a specific action is detected in the body or in the environment. Others are simply made on a set cycle. Our bodies make lots of hormones that have a wide variety of roles. Oestrogen is made by the ovaries and adrenaline is made by nerve cells and adrenal glands, which live on top of our kidneys. Hormones can make our hearts beat faster, make puberty happen, cause our bones to thicken with calcium or even send us to sleep.

Oxytocin plays an important role in the bonding a baby experiences soon after birth, and can even act as a kind of signalling mechanism between mother and baby. This hormone is produced by all of us, male and female, throughout our lives. It is a kind of social hormone. When we feel good, it is produced. And when our bodies are teeming with oxytocin, we feel even better.

Until recently it was believed that oxytocin was primarily related to having babies and feeding them. As researchers are discovering more about oxytocin we have begun to appreciate its important role in our overall physical health. Our hearts benefit greatly from this 'super' hormone. Oxytocin is released from the pituitary gland in both men and women in response to touch, during sex and in social bonding. Not just romantic bonding, by the way. It keeps us feeling linked to our friends and families too.

Research has found that oxytocin has several benefits for the heart. Oxytocin can prevent damage to a healthy heart and keep it healthy. We understand this happens in a couple of ways. Firstly, oxytocin can fight inflammation. Inflammation occurs when our bodies are sick or injured, and is a sign that our cells are fighting infection or trying to stop or repair damage from an injury. It's an important defence mechanism in our bodies. Inflammation can get carried away though and add to the damage. When the heart becomes inflamed after a heart attack or an infection, oxytocin may help limit the collateral damage done by inflammation.

Oxytocin can also affect a number of body systems directly linked to the heart. It causes blood vessels to relax, which enables the heart to pump more easily against the bigger vessels, as opposed to when the vessels are smaller and narrower. This also helps lower blood pressure, which is very important for getting blood to all the other vital organs like the kidneys and brain. Finally, oxytocin may also help heal injuries by assisting the body to grow new blood vessels to bring nutrients to an injured area.

Does this mean we should all order a top-up of oxytocin? Well, yes and no. Oxytocin is used as a medicine, sometimes called Pitocin or Syntocinon, to help induce childbirth. But while we're still in the early stages of discovering how useful oxytocin can be, the best way of obtaining a fix is via the old-fashioned route: by loving others and giving hugs freely to help release this feel-good hormone.

There are many other hormones strongly linked to the emotion of love. For instance, adrenaline is released when we're excited to see someone, especially when we're just getting to know them. Dopamine is a hormone that activates the parts of the brain that feel reward and help us to feel happy. Vasopressin is another hormone released from the same part of the brain as oxytocin and the two can work together, but sometimes vasopressin can antagonise oxytocin. It's a complex system that ebbs and flows. What's important about all of the hormones that are produced by love is that they make our bodies and cells feel good, and that ultimately makes us healthier.

Danielle's story

I met a patient once who was very young to be in the care of heart surgeons. In her mid-thirties, this woman had had a heart attack. A combination of genes and diabetes led her to develop coronary artery disease with bad blockages of her blood vessels. Her heart was at such risk that we kept her in hospital until she had her operation, connected to a drip to keep her blood vessels wide open and free from the sludge of blood clots.

Understandably, facing open-heart surgery can make you assess your life in ways you never thought possible. This patient was no different and so she requested that we put her operation on hold until she married her long-time partner. Her family swung into action, arranging a wedding in the ward. The bride would have to carry her drip stand down the aisle, which would be the bright corridor of the heart surgery ward.

Two days after her wedding she was wheeled down the same corridor to the operating theatre. Just like her wedding, the operation went off without a hitch. Of course, it takes more than a wedding for surgery to be successful, but I can't help but think that it didn't hurt that she had just married the love of her life. It may be speculation, but opposing all the stress hormones and heart disease was the flush of love-related hormones, putting her in the best possible frame of mind and physical condition.

Plus one

For many of us, the relationship we have with our partner is one of the most important in our lives. It is an interaction of romance, trust and companionship. A healthy relationship can provide so much to us socially and psychologically, but it also has a profound effect on our physical health.

Love, like any other emotion we feel, doesn't just occur in the mind. The mind and the brain are inextricably linked to the rest of the body. Love creates a cascade of changes, starting in the **limbic system**, which is our emotional powerhouse tucked away deep in our brains. When the limbic system fires off with love, the cascade carries through the body, reducing stress both in the brain and the body, and allows us to develop a kind of social and psychological resistance. It feeds back on itself, growing stronger, and we grow stronger too.

When we feel love, the emotion that triggers the limbic system also sends messages to our nerves, telling them to relax us. Our heart rate and blood pressure drop as oxytocin and other hormone messengers relax our blood vessels. Parts of our brain called 'reward centres' fire up, telling our bodies that we are pretty pleased with what's going on, and the cycle repeats, getting stronger. When we are loved, we sometimes describe how we 'melt', and on the inside the love is melting away stress, anxiety and physical pain. It is an apt metaphor and describes the beauty of the body's response better than any words of medicine or science ever could.

All of these reactions are good for us, both when we are ill and when we are healthy – to prevent us from becoming ill. While the body may be experiencing all of these valuable benefits, does it make us well? Can love heal?

Most studies in this area look specifically at marriage for historical reasons – marriage was more common than de facto–type relationships in the past. It's also easier to research details such as whether someone was married or not from databases that collect information on health and death. Although we're talking about marriage, the social and biological advantages of marriage extend beyond its legal status and are used as a marker of long-term relationships.

In the past, whether or not someone was married would not have been considered a significant factor in a person's health or recovery from illness. We now have scientific evidence showing how important being in a relationship is for your health, and when it comes to hearts, it's even more so.

When we look at patients who have heart disease, those who are married tend to recover better than those who are not. This is particularly the case for men. Some scientific studies report rates of dying as around double in men who are on their own. Interestingly though, in polygamous societies it has been found that having more than one wife is bad for a man's heart health.

Strangely, women who are married don't experience the same protective effect. While they are more likely to recover better than widowed or unmarried women, the health benefits for men are much more pronounced. It's not clear why, but it may be that women try to return to their pre-heart-attack ways of looking after everyone else. It might also be that women who have heart disease are more ill from their disease than men. Either way, when we look at all the reasons people may have health problems, having a plus one is better for their health.

It's not just traditional marriage between a man and a woman that has been found to have health benefits. Same-sex marriage is also good for health. People who are LGBTIQ have much worse health outcomes than heterosexual people, but when we look at what happens to people in same-sex marriages, their health improves, with less psychological illness. In the United States, legalising same-sex marriage gave many spouses access to healthcare plans and insurance, which meant that people were potentially able to access preventative care or seek healthcare earlier than they previously could.

Before we get to the stage of being ill though, prevention is exceptionally important, and this is another area in which men seem to significantly benefit from marriage. Married men tend to shy away from habits that are bad for them, like smoking or drinking too much, and they carry less weight. They are also more likely to see their doctors for prevention. While all couples will to some degree benefit in a social way from marriage, wives seem to be instrumental in keeping their husbands' health a priority.

It makes sense that the love and security provided by marriage or a stable relationship are important. There also seems to be a link between the quality of a relationship and the health benefits that follow. Some studies have looked at the effects of relationships on inflammation. Incredibly, being in a stable and satisfied relationship reduces the amount of inflammation that our body has to deal with on a daily basis.

If you have a furry plus one in your life, that is another valuable way to give and receive love. Having a pet can fire up all of those good parts of the brain and hormones that help to heal your body and fight disease. Just as importantly, pets can make you feel physically and mentally better.

Can we love ourselves to better health?

Loving ourselves is all the rage and is central to all kinds of advice we receive on seeking happiness and health. We must love ourselves before anyone else will love us. We must love ourselves to be physically and mentally healthy. We should work out because we love our bodies, not because we hate them. Self-love and self-compassion are gaining huge amounts of attention lately, especially for women, perhaps to fight the unrelenting standards placed on how we should look, behave, exercise or what we should wear. It's prescribed as the perfect balance to the perfect life we should be striving for.

Self-compassion is a wonderful term to describe a process of loving yourself. It is a real psychological and social phenomenon, not just a hashtag. It's about maintaining a positive, compassionate attitude towards yourself, even when faced with your own failures or shortcomings. It's about being kind to yourself when you fail to meet whatever goal or benchmark you have set. Self-compassion is understanding that your behaviour often happens in the face of difficulties. You're aware that you are not alone, and you realise that it's hard for everyone else too. You are not holding yourself to an unrealistic ideal, and you are able to look at your negative emotions without feeling as though everything is crashing down. It's about not buying into the catastrophe or dwelling on the overwhelming disaster of your emotion, but just acknowledging that it's there.

Self-compassion is not self-esteem. Self-esteem often relies on comparing how you're doing with other people. Self-compassion is about working on your emotions and opinions towards yourself and recognising that they drive your biology and behaviour.

Self-compassion is great in situations when you feel that you may not be deserving of kindness. Cultivating self-compassion enables you to develop the tools to manage when times are tough. Think of it as training for a grand final: you are not going to obtain the best result if you just turn up to the game. But if you train throughout the season, it's just another game.

So many aspects of our lives and emotions are directly connected in our bodies. Emotional states and the biological processes that they influence in the body can dictate our behaviour negatively or positively. Thinking back to the marriage effect on men's health, aside from the direct physical benefits of feeling love and support, some of the positive effects are due to the fact that men are more likely to engage in healthy behaviours when they are married. They smoke and drink less and keep a healthier body weight. Self-compassion has a similar effect, mostly on eating and weight loss.

If you are too hard on yourself and lack compassion, it can affect your body image. Studies have demonstrated that young women who are dissatisfied with their bodies and eat poorly because of it (too much or too little) may lack the ability to soothe themselves; in other words, they are unable to discard negative self-talk or be more accepting of their flaws. It sounds like something that we teach babies, but adults need it too. Studies have shown that these women may have brains that are constantly on high alert looking for problems in themselves and around them. This sets them up to be perfectionists, but not in a good way. This kind of perfectionism may mean that while they're being so hard on themselves, they're also not taking care of or loving their bodies.

Many of us struggle with our weight, and since exercising and eating are behaviours, other behaviours, like self-compassion, can impact on the ability to maintain a healthy weight or lose weight. Research has tracked young men and women over many years, looking at their weight and matching that with how they felt about themselves. It found that women who had poor self-esteem or self-image were more likely to be heavier than those who didn't.

Interestingly, this didn't always seem true for men. This tendency also didn't track as strongly the older they became.

At times when we might try to look our best or stay in shape – for instance, when we're dating – we correspondingly feel more attractive and confident in our appearance. This feeling of confidence is strongest during these times and feeds back positively into our opinion of ourselves. This is then reflected in our behaviour, self-esteem and, most importantly, our health.

What I find fascinating about this topic are the ways in which we exert self-kindness or self-compassion. Sometimes we can prioritise how we feel over our health. The old story of a heartbroken woman alone with a spoon and a tub of ice cream to soothe herself is a cliché, yet has a ring of truth. Most of us have justified a chocolate binge, another cigarette or a big night out drinking as a form of being kind to ourselves, blowing away life's troubles with calories, nicotine or alcohol. While at its heart this kind of behaviour could be considered a form of self-kindness or compassion, it's not something that promotes health.

That's why it's important to develop self-soothing, self-compassion tools that don't rely on anyone else or on junk food or alcohol to fix a problem. Self-compassion behaviours that we can practise and develop to use at the end of a bad day at work, or after a fight with our partner, or a slip in a diet, can be useful and healthy.

Love heals all?

The idea that the power of love can heal disease is a beautiful one. Unfortunately, the science is not conclusive. What we do know is that marriage has a positive effect on heart health, especially for men. It's just a marker though for happiness and healthy behaviours. When it comes to self-compassion or, colloquially, loving yourself, the picture is even less clear.

The science of love, whether it is love for someone else or for yourself, is still under consideration. In the world of science, love may heal, but to be honest, we don't know for sure. We can say with some certainty that the opposite of being loved and cared for – that is, being isolated and sad – puts your heart at risk.

Love is an area of emotional and physical health that ties our minds and bodies together in ways we don't quite understand. As we learn more about the heart and the effect of our emotions on it, the pathways and biology of these processes may become clearer. For the time being though, love is good for our minds, our social development and probably our bodies, to a degree. It is a medicine that we should give and seek freely.

chapter 6
FEEDING YOUR HEART

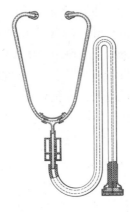

One cannot think well, love well, sleep well, if one has not dined well
VIRGINIA WOOLF, WRITER

Food is an enormously important part of our lives. It's integral to the ways we socialise and is used to celebrate occasions and bond families and friendships. Cooking for a loved one is seen as an act of care. Food is also a treat, a reward for a job well done. We love it so much that the world now has more disease from an excess of food than a lack of food.

You might be shocked to learn that nutrition is not taught well in medical school. My education on nutrition basically consisted of an in-depth discussion of breastfeeding that culminated in equating drinking cow's milk with drinking breast milk. It's probably not surprising then that over the years I have followed many questionable diets that offered minimal nutrition or calories and a good deal of suffering. Just like a lot of the population.

Since leaving medical school and beginning work in a field that is often intrinsically tied to problems stemming from what we eat, I have made a point of learning about food and how it makes us sick. As a doctor, I have never considered it was adequate advice to simply tell patients to 'eat better'. After all, what does that look like? And how do we do it? I confess that I love food, including food that is bad for me! What and how we eat is such a complex social, biological and psychological process, there is so much to unravel in order to make good choices.

The evidence that being overweight is unhealthy for you is quite literally everywhere. Everyone from doctors to Instagrammers to your mother is telling you what to eat and when. Despite this, it's nearly impossible to know for certain what you should eat for optimal health.

As nutrition science evolves, we learn more about how what we feed ourselves influences our ability to fight disease. Calorie counting used to be a staple of dieters, but now we are learning that the quality, not just the quantity, of food that we eat has direct effects on health.

The heart is affected by our diet in numerous ways, but probably the most important effects relate to our coronary arteries. As we've learnt, coronary arteries that become blocked cause heart attacks or angina, a precursor to a heart attack. These blockages are caused by plaque swelling out from the vessel walls. They have large amounts of cholesterol in them, a kind of fat that we obtain from food. When this discovery was made, fat became a target for heart disease crusaders. Diets and tablets were developed to lower the amount of fat and cholesterol circulating in our bloodstreams.

Since those early days our understanding of fats in the blood and body has increased rapidly, but the role of fats, and which diets and drugs can be helpful, has been subject to debate. Irrespective of any new knowledge, obesity, diabetes and high blood fats are all still associated with heart disease and are toxic to our hearts. So what can we do about that?

Obesity

Several years ago we operated on a young woman in her forties. She had such severe blockages in her heart arteries that she had dreadful chest pain even walking around her home. She weighed around 140 kilograms and was what might be called morbidly obese. It's not a pretty term, but basically it means that a person is carrying so much extra weight in the form of fat that they are highly susceptible to life-threatening diseases and complications. Her heart disease was one of those complications.

This woman's surgery went well; she had two bypass grafts to her blocked arteries and her angina went away. She recovered reasonably well, a little slowly because she hadn't walked very much due to her chest pain, but she recuperated. One morning we went to visit her on our ward round. In addition to her one piece of toast from the hospital breakfast she had somehow scored an extra six pieces, all piled high and spread with butter. She'd asked the meal service staff for extras and had donations from other patients who weren't keen on theirs.

We know that shame is a terrible motivator when it comes to changing behaviour. That doesn't mean that frustration doesn't get the better of all of us from time to time. One of the doctors on the team was infuriated and proceeded to tell her that she would never get well if she didn't stop eating herself to death. He looked at her, exasperated, and said, 'You've had heart surgery, open-heart surgery. How can that not be enough to make you want to change?' The tone was not helpful but it did, in my mind, raise an important question. Why can't we lose weight, even when our hearts depend on it?

Obesity has been declared public health enemy number one and sits atop lists of public health issues that governments and health organisations like the World Health Organisation want to address. The proportion of obese children and adults worldwide continues to grow. Since the early 1980s rates of obesity have roughly doubled around the world. Diseases of excess food or calorie consumption are now overtaking diseases of under-nutrition, even in developing countries.

Over two-thirds of the populations of the United States and Australia are now considered overweight or obese. While carrying extra weight tends to make the news when plane seats are at stake, what is lacking attention is that most of the top 10 causes of death are associated with obesity, such as heart disease, strokes and some cancers. The endless availability of calorie-dense foods, large servings, doing less physical activity at home and at work, and the tendency to spend more time on sedentary activities like watching TV or using computers, are making us fat. Essentially we expend less energy but consume more. When we have an excess of energy, our body stores it for later use and this leads to weight gain.

Going back to my patient, how did she get to that point? Basically she ate more than her body needed for the level of activity she did. That is a simple maths equation, and as nice and tidy as that is, life isn't like that and neither is diet. Humans are a fascinating and complex mix of our genes, our environment, our emotions, the processes within our bodies and much more. Although gaining weight is as simple as not enough output for too much intake, the reality is that obesity occurs in a complex set of circumstances.

DNA and genes act as a blueprint for how our bodies are built and operated, and when it comes to the likelihood of being overweight, our genes can cause trouble. Heritability is the proportion our genes contribute to a certain trait, such as eye colour, height or weight. In the case of body weight, years of scientific study have led us to understand that somewhere between 40 and 70 per cent of how our bodies carry weight is determined by our genes. A very small proportion of people who are overweight or obese have defective single genes that promote weight gain.

Even if we're genetically predisposed to being bigger, that's not the only way that we wind up overweight. Our brains and bodies use a complex system of nerves and hormones that regulate our appetite, how much we eat and what happens to it. The hypothalamus is in the centre of the brain and when the nerve cells in that area are bathed in hormones they can make us eat less or more. Other parts of our bodies, like our fat cells, stomachs and even the bugs that live in our guts, send out signals that affect how we eat. For some of us, when we diet or lose weight, these signals can go into overdrive, which is one of the many reasons it's easy to regain weight.

Added to this is the environment we live in. Calorie-dense food tastes good and is pleasurable to eat. Stress can encourage eating, both due to the body's basic need to gain energy in times of crisis and because we have learnt to see food as comfort. This interplay, and how it affects weight loss and weight management, makes obesity a difficult and chronic disease.

It's important to think of obesity and being overweight as a disease, not a social phenomenon, a fashion faux pas or a moral error. Most of the weight we gain in the form of fat is stored in the subcutaneous area, under the skin. That's the rolls on our stomachs or hips or wherever we tend to store extra fat. Most of this fat is made up of **triglycerides**, which have been strongly linked with creating the plaque that blocks coronary arteries in heart disease. The fat cells aren't alone though; they are joined by a number of cells from the immune system, and between them they make special kinds of molecules that cause inflammation in the body. As we've seen, inflammation can be useful in healing, but when it's left unchecked, it makes us prone to diseases like heart disease.

Visceral fat isn't the type of fat that makes your clothes fit badly. 'Viscera' is a Latin-derived word for organs. In this type of fat storage the fat surrounds your vital organs – such as your heart, liver, kidneys and pancreas. It might sound cosy to cuddle your organs in a layer of insulation, but the fat around these organs almost strangles them. This kind of fat has been shown to cause high blood pressure when it surrounds the kidneys. It is also linked to diabetes and fatty liver, and can promote plaque build-up in the blood vessels. Just like fat under the skin, this kind of fat makes molecules that cause unnecessary inflammation and harm the way your organs function.

Holding on to extra fat is literally toxic to the heart. Being overweight is associated with conditions that pose serious risks to the heart, such as diabetes and high blood pressure. Research has shown that fat is a metabolically active tissue, meaning that it has a wide variety of functions. When it comes to the heart, the hormones that fat produces aggravate the inside of the blood vessels and may even directly injure the heart muscle. Fatty tissue also activates other hormones and nerve pathways to cause high blood pressure and injury to the blood vessels, paving the way for developing plaque called **atheroma** that blocks the vital arteries.

Can you be fit and fat?

If you're carrying extra weight, is it possible to be fit and healthy? It's a question I'm asked frequently. And it's a pretty tough one to answer, to be honest. On one hand, the science of carrying extra weight, especially around your organs, tells us that if you are heavier than what is deemed a healthy weight, even if you can run a marathon, your health may be at risk. On the other hand, weight or body mass index (BMI) are pretty blunt instruments when it comes to measuring health, and they don't tell us exactly where you are carrying extra weight or if it's definitely unhealthy.

A small proportion of people who are considered overweight or obese (as determined by BMI) can still be healthy and not suffer from diabetes or high blood pressure. This can only be determined by a doctor and by having blood lipids (cholesterol and its close cousins), blood sugar and blood pressure checked.

In short, you can be heavier and fit; you may even still be healthy. For some, determining that from weight alone is like trying to read a book in the dark. However, since science confirms that keeping off extra fat is definitely good for you, it follows that you should strive as best you can for a healthy body weight and minimise the fat you carry.

A little weight loss goes a long way

Most people are aware that losing weight is hard and part of that difficulty comes from the way our bodies react when we lose weight. Our bodies can sometimes send the same signals to eat and store energy even when we've lost weight. Over time these signals can go away, but because our bodies fight diets, even after losing weight it's important to keep managing obesity as if it were still there.

The health benefits of losing weight, especially to the heart, are huge. Even losing five per cent of your starting weight can improve the way your pancreas handles sugars. In studies of people who lost five to 10 per cent of their body weight, the resulting decrease in blood pressure, cholesterol and blood sugar was enough to reduce their risk of high blood pressure and diabetes. People with these conditions can in a sense be 'cured' by losing weight through diet and exercise or surgery. Some are even able to stop taking medicines as a result.

Our society is obsessed with beauty and being slim, often solely for appearance's sake. In reality, much more important than washboard abs or a small dress size is being a healthy weight. We need to be aware of the huge favour we do our insides by even a five per cent weight loss. Looking after our bodies is the most beautiful thing we can do for ourselves.

BMI – hot or not?

BMI stands for body mass index and is calculated by dividing your weight in kilograms by your height squared in metres. What you are left with is a two-digit number that is your BMI. Your BMI then falls into one of these categories:

* Normal 18.5–24.9
* Overweight 25–29.9
* Obese 30–34.9
* Severely obese 35–39.9
* Morbidly obese – over 40

BMI receives plenty of criticism, much of it fair. Weight is a crude tool and doesn't account for what that weight is made up of (fat or muscle) or where it's found (around your stomach, organs or hips). So it may incorrectly classify someone who is shorter with more muscle, for example. Likewise, if you fall into the healthy category, you may still carry fat around your organs, which is not healthy. It may also be misleading for racial groups with different body compositions to Caucasians.

So why do we use it? It does seem to correlate with health outcomes when we look at large groups of people. For example, a higher BMI is associated with heart attacks at a younger age. It's also an easy test to calculate. However, as a predictor of health outcomes for the general population, a measurement such as waist-to-hip ratio may be a better tool. To calculate this ratio, measure your waist and then your hips, and if the ratio is greater than 1.0 in men or 0.85 in women, your heart needs some extra love, pronto.

Cholesterol: public enemy number one?

I was in the supermarket, browsing through the cold section that houses the milk and cheese. I was after some butter, which may sound terrible with some of the dietary advice around. (Regardless of that, a bit of butter probably isn't the worst food you can put in your body.) There were butters and margarines and spreads as far as the eye could see. Some with low salt, some with flavour, some with no fat. And then I noticed a special 'spread' that claimed to reduce cholesterol. Magic butter perhaps?

Cholesterol is inevitably mentioned when we discuss heart health. Your doctor might order a cholesterol test as part of a regular health check and you will need to address your cholesterol if it is found to be 'too high'. Despite all the talk, we don't tend to explain exactly what cholesterol is and why it's important.

Cholesterol is a vital part of our bodies. It's a type of lipid or fat molecule that is an important component in the tiny walls that make up all of our cells. Our bodies also need cholesterol to make bile (the green liquid our gall bladder stores that helps our gut deal with fats we eat) and to make vitamin D. Essentially, no animals can live without cholesterol. Our bodies can make cholesterol, mainly in the liver. We also get it from our diet, predominantly from animal sources like meat, egg yolks, milk and cheese.

The fact that cholesterol is vital for life does not mean it is always healthy: you can have too much of a good thing. When we talk about 'cholesterol' generically, we're usually talking about three separate molecules. Cholesterol is like a group of cousins, including high-density lipoprotein (HDL) and low-density lipoprotein (LDL), and all are involved in forming plaque inside our arteries. LDL is sometimes called 'bad cholesterol'. It circulates around the body, away from places it can be excreted, like the liver, but close to places where it can cause mischief, namely in the blood vessels.

When a blood vessel is injured (from age, smoking, diabetes or our genes) these bad cholesterol molecules rush to the scene and invade the blood vessel wall, making it swell. Our bodies then call in other cells like platelets, muscle cells and immune cells to try to help, but they only make plaque that can block the artery. This is called **atherosclerosis**, which means 'fatty scar'. It's what is responsible for heart attacks and strokes.

HDL is sometimes called 'good cholesterol'. The reason HDL is good for us is that it basically does the opposite of LDL by pulling together the bad cholesterols from around the body (including plaque in our arteries). They're sent to the liver where they're turned into bile, stored in the gall bladder and then pushed into the bowel where, well, they are gotten rid of in our poo.

Scientific studies show a very strong link between higher cholesterol levels and heart disease. At the same time, other clinical trials give slightly different findings – that cholesterol and LDL in the blood may reduce the risk of heart disease. Despite the differences, most trials that look at the benefit of lowering cholesterol and LDL show that heart attacks are reduced by somewhere between 19 and 34 per cent, which by medical standards is a big drop after treating just one risk factor.

The association of cholesterol with heart disease has come under intense scrutiny in recent times, with vocal opponents stating that we have been misled. They say it's not cholesterol that causes blockages in our arteries but sugar, inflammation or other culprits. Scientific evidence on cholesterol is not perfect, but it is strong enough to confirm that it has a role. I agree that a number of other factors are at play, such as sugar and hormonal patterns.

But to let cholesterol off the hook based on the current evidence seems premature.

Fats

In 2015 the US Departments of Agriculture and Health released the Dietary Guidelines for Americans. For the first time ever the guidelines did not tell Americans how much fat they should eat. The recommended fat intake used to be around 25 to 30 per cent of total calorie consumption, as fat was viewed as the primary reason people were getting bigger and sicker. These guidelines echoed an emerging trend. Rather than promoting restriction, they promoted choosing good, healthy food, including healthy fat. This was a change from recommending that everything eaten should be low fat.

Scientific evidence has found that not all fats are created equal. And this has profound implications for the way we view fats and their impact on heart disease. Fats are classified according to chemical composition, how long a chain of individual fatty acids is and how they're joined together by chemical bonds. Saturated fats are found in animal meats and dairy, plant oils like coconut oil and palm oil, and most commercially made foods like cakes or doughnuts. Trans fatty acids (sometimes called trans fats) occur in beef, lamb and dairy, and in a chemical change in vegetable oils called partial hydrogenation. Partially hydrogenated vegetable oils are produced in factories to make oil-based products more spreadable. Polyunsaturated fatty acids, such as linoleic acid and those found in fish, are long chains of fatty acids that have a vital role in the production of a number of hormones in our bodies. Monounsaturated fatty acids are those found in nuts and olive oil.

The classification is important, not just because these molecules look alike but because their effects on our health can be similar.

Saturated fats, for example, originally received most of the blame for causing heart disease by raising bad cholesterol levels. It may not be as cut and dried as we once thought, though: the link between saturated fats and heart disease has since been questioned. Despite this, a recent large study by the American Heart Association confirmed the link, but also recommended replacing saturated fat with polyunsaturated fat. What we replace saturated fat with in our diets may also be worse for us than the saturated fat itself. There is more investigation to be done on fats, and I'm sure we will see further debate.

The same study came down hard on coconut oil. Coconut oil is enjoying time in the limelight, with claims it is a 'superfood' with significant health benefits, including reducing the risk of heart disease. Despite this, it is extremely high in saturated fat. In a number of scientific studies looking at how coconut oil impacts the amount of fats and cholesterol in our blood, coconut oil had an inconsistent effect on cholesterol. It tended to increase LDL cholesterol (bad cholesterol) overall, and this was not offset with enough beneficial effects to make consuming it worthwhile.

The two unsaturated fat groups, polyunsaturated and mono-unsaturated fats, are often called 'good fats'. To be perfectly frank, labelling any foods or nutrients as 'good' or 'bad' fails to recognise the complexity of our bodies and the foods themselves. However, unsaturated fats may be incredibly useful at directly fighting some of the processes that result in heart disease. Foods containing these types of fats can increase HDL cholesterol, reduce inflammation, improve the way our bodies handle sugar and insulin, and help blood flow smoothly through our blood vessels.

The last group, trans fats, is likely to be where problems arise. Even though trans fats are found in small amounts in natural, unprocessed foods, we have started eating much more of this type of fat. As food manufacturers realised how useful trans fats were at preventing food from spoiling and making naturally solid foods spreadable, their production and use skyrocketed. The trade-off for margarine that spreads nicely on toast is that we consume too much of a fat that is bad news. Trans fats don't just increase our risk of heart disease, they also impede our body's ability to obtain beneficial effects from unsaturated fats. Trans fats have been implicated in increased rates of obesity, type 2 diabetes, some types of cancer and even Alzheimer's disease. The US Food and Drug Administration (FDA) has mandated that trans fats be given the flick from all foods.

For years, fats and cholesterol were viewed as 'bad'. Now, we don't seem to know. Fat may be good, and what we replace it with may be bad. Chemical modification of fats (trans fats) may poison us. What does this fat science mean? The first point to remember is that nutrition and clinical science have evolved greatly in the last decade or so, and will continue to do so for years to come. This may sound like bad news, because this whole fat thing is exhausting enough already. Realistically, though, newer information is simply displacing older, less helpful information, which can only be a good thing.

The second point to keep in mind is this: the fat that makes the zips on our jeans tight and the number on the scales higher may still be good for our health. It doesn't just come from butter, meat and oil. Fat stored in our bodies is the end result of having to pack away extra energy that we ate and did not need. The fat that we consume in our diet is different and may not make us bigger; in fact some of it may make us healthier.

What does this science tell us about how to look after ourselves? Just like the complexities of the different fats, foods containing fat aren't all equal when it comes to our health. Red meat, for example, contains macronutrients (like protein and fat) as well as micronutrients (like iron) that are good for us – the key is whether or not it is processed. Eating unprocessed red meat doesn't appear to cause heart disease. However, if we eat it in a fast-food burger or in some other kind of processed food (meat pie anyone?) it does increase our risk of heart disease. Early research suggests that animal products such as dairy and eggs, which have been considered unhealthy for years, may in fact make our hearts healthier. A word of caution though: the data used to make this assumption is still being studied.

The well-known Mediterranean Diet is rich in fish, vegetables, nuts and healthy oils and is consistently associated with good heart health. Virgin olive oil, an integral part of this diet, contains monounsaturated fatty acids. When it is refined to remove colour or flavour, its health benefits may be compromised. Cooking with virgin olive oil strongly reduces the risk of heart disease and stroke. Nuts are another food that we were cautioned against eating in years gone by. They are rich in polyunsaturated and monounsaturated fats as well as containing a number of minerals and vitamins. More recently, large trials found that people who ate nuts regularly decreased their cholesterol levels (especially the LDL levels) in as little as 24 weeks. Other trials have shown that people who ate nuts four or more times per week reduced their risk of heart disease.

Some food and supplements that were once believed, anecdotally at least, to be helpful in treating high cholesterol have been proven to have no benefits at all. In some cases they may even cause harm. One such case is coconut oil, which may raise LDL cholesterol (bad cholesterol) levels. Garlic is another dietary treatment that, despite claims, fails to make a difference, as are supplements like red yeast rice and selenium. Eating a diet high in foods like olive oil, fish, nuts and other unprocessed forms of fat is a better first step. Following this, a plant-based diet, including plenty of fruits and vegetables, is the safest way forward.

Sugar

When you are 94 years young, as one of my patients puts it, people listen to what you have to say. Particularly when you've lived a healthy life – your opinion on good health matters. This patient is a dynamite woman who in her forties won a healthy-eating prize for her commitment to eating fresh, healthful foods. The strictest food rule in her household? No sugar. This meant no juice, no soft drink, no lollies – just meat, fruit and vegetables. In fact, her eldest son bought a bottle of Coke with his first pay packet, a treat that was never in the household when he was growing up.

Sugar is now firmly in the crosshairs when it comes to healthy eating. Major health agencies, including the World Health Organisation, have stated that no more than 10 per cent of energy intake should come from sugar. Other agencies, such as Public Health England, have stated that it should be five per cent. It's an interesting change, considering these kinds of recommendations used to be made regarding dietary fat.

The average amount of sugar consumed on a daily basis has grown dramatically in developed countries in recent years. Most of this increase has come from sugar added to foods we eat, not in naturally occurring sources such as fruit or milk. The evidence linking this increase with heart disease, diabetes, some cancers and obesity is damning. Research into the effects of sugar on heart health has in many instances focused on sugar-sweetened beverages (soft drink, fizzy drink or soda, depending on where you come from). This research has confirmed that the more of these drinks we consume, the worse it is for our health.

A study looking at how many American adults consumed more than the recommended sugar intake of 10 per cent per day found that over 70 per cent of the thousands of people studied missed the mark. Around 10 per cent of people ate more than a quarter of their daily food intake in sugar. What was incredibly frightening about this was not just how much sugar people consumed but what it meant for their health. Consuming between 10 and 25 per cent of calories in sugar meant that the risk of dying from heart disease was around 1.5 times more than for those who ate less than 10 per cent. And the heavy-hitters of 25 per cent or more? Their risk was as high as 3.5 times greater!

Where is all of this sugar coming from? We're not just sitting down at the table with a bowl of sugar; this sugar is hidden away in sugar-sweetened drinks, fruit drinks, desserts and candy. Sugar-sweetened drinks are particularly nasty and a number of studies have taken aim at Coke and other soft drinks as being a big factor in why we're becoming bigger and sicker. Even when we take into account other problems known to be bad for our hearts, like cholesterol and blood pressure, these cans of sugar cause damage independent of those.

How is sugar causing all of this mischief? First of all, it's important to understand that, like fat, not all sugars are created equal. Most interest is focused on two types of sugar: sucrose and fructose. Sucrose is a disaccharide, which means it is two separate sugars, bonded together. The two sugars are glucose and fructose, in equal shares. It's basically the table sugar that we put in our coffees or in our baking.

Fructose is found naturally in honey, fruit and some vegetables, and is added to many commercially available foods and drinks in the form of high-fructose corn syrup. It's made of more fructose than glucose and is cheap to produce, which is why companies use it to sweeten foods. Fructose seems to be unlike other sugars in the way it affects the body.

The liver is the super-intelligent organ responsible for waste (as well as a number of other important functions we won't go into here). It receives fat, sugar, drugs and all kinds of compounds in the body. The liver processes the fat and sugar from foods we eat. When fructose floats through the liver, just like with other compounds, the liver pushes it through a series of chemical reactions, ultimately making substrates for energy that can be used directly by our cells or stored in the form of fat. Unlike glucose though, fructose can act as the base molecule for the liver to produce triglycerides, a form of fat. The liver works very hard to process all of this fructose and starts to make by-products like uric acid, which can be toxic to blood vessels and cells.

When we eat or drink fructose, our cholesterol levels skyrocket. LDL cholesterol, triglycerides and uric acid can be measured at very high levels in people who consume large amounts of unnatural fructose. They also tend to secrete large amounts of insulin from the pancreas, which prompts the body to store extra energy as fat. Blood tests show that hormones associated with inflammation rise with the consumption of foods or drinks high in fructose, and this in turn can cause blood vessels to become inflamed and injured. What's more, these sugar-filled beverages don't satisfy our appetites, so we eat more calories to feel full.

You may have noted that I skipped over the fact that fructose is contained in fruit. Does that mean that we should give up fruit to avoid dangerous fructose? Absolutely not! Fruit has incredible health benefits and to consume the amount of fructose that would be comparable to drinking a can of Coke, you'd have to eat huge amounts of fruit. Unlike soft drink, fruit is filling because it contains fibre and is rich in other nutrients, including vitamins and minerals.

Public health organisations are recommending we reduce the amount of sugars, particularly fructose, we consume by limiting the number of sugar-sweetened beverages we drink. Replacing a can of Coke with water is the preferred strategy. It has been found that over the course of a year, people who swap water for soft drink gain around half a kilo less than they would if they drank soft drink. It also dramatically drops the risk of developing diabetes, which would have to be one of the biggest threats to our health.

Aside from skipping the can of soft drink, how else can we avoid sugar? The easiest way is to avoid processed foods. Most processed foods are all about taste and less about nutrition. The good taste of modern food often comes from added sugars, frequently in the form of high-fructose corn syrup.

When it comes to artificial sweeteners, the jury is still out. While drinking or eating foods that aren't sweetened with sugar might seem like a good idea, the longer-term effects of artificial sweeteners aren't well known yet. Some research has suggested that diet drinks can trick the body into creating fat even without the sugar. Other studies have drawn an early link to problems with the liver, bones and even our brains. Like much of nutrition science, this is an area of growing research: watch this space.

Bugs! The gut microbiome

We are covered in bugs. They are on our skin and up our noses, but by far the winner when it comes to bug numbers is the gut. It's estimated there are more than 100 trillion bugs living in or on our bodies, most of them in the large intestine. Far from being problematic, our lives depend on them. They are dependent on us to survive too. We have a symbiotic relationship.

This is not news though. We've known we're teeming with bacteria for many years. However, in recent times we're learning more and more about just how important these bugs are for our health. The host of bugs that live in the gut is called the microbiome, basically a large city of different bacteria. Its role is to help with digestion and prevent disease by drowning out bad bacteria. The make-up of this city of bugs is extremely important and has far-reaching effects beyond keeping our colon healthy. In fact, the health of the gut microbiome is important for organs throughout the body, including the brain and the heart.

Gut microbes are our first line of defence against the unhealthy food and drinks we eat. The bugs that make up each person's microbiome are different. If two people were to eat the same meal, their bodies may process it entirely differently depending on the bugs that live in their colons. This is exciting because it means we can influence which bugs live in the colon, and we may be able to encourage the gut to grab the good nutrients and let go of the bad. For our hearts, influencing those bacteria could mean we are capable of exposing our hearts to mainly good nutrients, discarding anything that is 'bad' for them.

The individual types of bugs that live in the colon can create molecules from the foods that we eat, particularly when it comes to fats and sugars. These molecules can harm us or help us. If the wrong bacteria produce the wrong molecules, our blood can become thicker and more likely to block vital arteries in the heart. This can also cause cholesterol to be soaked up into our blood vessels, creating plaque, and can even impair our heart's ability to deal with injury. If we take away bacteria that may be protective in storing and processing sugars and fats, our risk of developing diabetes and obesity can increase.

So how can we change the bugs in our guts? One way would be a faecal transplant. Poo is made up of bacteria from our colon and if we take the bacteria of a person of normal weight with a healthy heart, and transplant it into a person who is overweight, that person may be able to lose weight. For day-to-day use, faecal transplants are not ideal, though. Another way to influence the good bacteria is to change what we eat in order to allow the good bugs to grow and the bad ones to go.

While we're busy eating trans fats and high-fructose corn syrup, we're missing out on vital nutrients that can help the good bacteria to triumph. One of the major nutrients that is beneficial to the gut bugs is fibre, which we find in fruit and vegetables or unrefined carbohydrates (whole grains). Eating these foods provides energy and makes the good bacteria healthy so that they can thrive. When we change this part of our diet, the way our liver processes sugar can be drastically altered and can reduce obesity and harmful fats in our blood stream, which in turn can fight disease and make our hearts happy and healthy.

chapter 7
EXERCISE: GETTING THAT HEART PUMPING

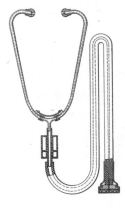

Lack of activity destroys the good condition of every human being, while movement and methodical physical exercise save it and preserve it
PLATO, GREEK PHILOSOPHER

I'm not what you would call a gifted athlete. To do OK at any given sport, I've always had to really slog it out. My brother, on the other hand, was one of those people who would pick up a bat or a racquet and just be great at it. It was infuriating. As I grew up though, I started to take up sport because I enjoyed it. I joined a running club and began training three times a week, heading out on weekends for a long run along the beautiful routes of Sydney. It was for my mind as much as my body.

I remember my first half marathon. I had trained hard and I was beyond excited. A girl who had always been mediocre at sport, I was about to run 21.1 kilometres. Around 16 kilometres into the race, everything started to hurt. This coincided with a big hill that hurt my mind as much as my body. At 18 kilometres, I was ready to throw my hands up and leave. At 21.1 kilometres, as I ran down the finishers' chute and saw people waving and cheering for me, I nearly cried with happiness. Clearly lacking blood supply to my brain, I wanted to run it again, right then. I suppose that's what they call a runner's high.

Given how exhausted I was at the end of this race, it would be reasonable to think that running 21.1 kilometres is not good for the heart. Not long after I completed this half marathon, I had an echocardiogram. It was an unusual experience to have my own heart scrutinised. An echocardiogram is an ultrasound of the heart to look at how it works and check it is pumping well and that all the parts are in order. As the technician looked at my heart, he asked whether I did much exercise. I immediately panicked, thinking he had found a problem, but what he had seen was a heart that was working extremely well due to all of the exercise I had been giving it. I breathed a sigh of relief and was thankful that, although running gave me sore legs, it had also given me a very strong heart.

There is no doubt that exercise is good for you. Exercise is so beneficial that the day after a patient has had heart surgery, we get them walking around the ward. People who have had a mechanical heart – an LVAD – inserted are told to work out at a gym at least three times a week once they leave hospital. I've watched the LVAD patients working out in our special cardiac gym and they put me to shame. In fact, every year a number of our transplant recipients and LVAD patients run or walk a local fun run, not only raising awareness of transplants but also doing their bodies a world of good.

When you exercise, sometimes it doesn't feel as if you're doing your heart any good. If you're anything like me, you go a nice shade of red, puff and pant up the hills, or wobble around as you try to hold warrior pose. You feel your heart race and when you're going hard, your lungs burn. Sweat drips and you wonder if you will make it back home. However, exercise is one of the best things you can do for your heart, your whole body and your mind, despite the puffing and panting.

Your heart on exercise

You've laced up your shoes and you're heading out the door. Whatever sport or exercise you choose, one thing is constant: your muscles are going to be doing extra work. When a part of your body needs to work harder, it needs more blood bringing it oxygen and glucose so that it can work faster and stronger.

One of the first things you notice when you exercise is that your heart rate jumps. At rest, say sitting down, most of us will have a heart rate of 60 to 80 beats per minute; women are usually a little higher than men. You can feel your pulse by pressing a few centimetres below your thumb at your radial artery or in your neck at the carotid artery. Some people who are very fit have resting heart rates as low as 30 to 40 beats per minute as their hearts have become very efficient.

When you start exercising, your heart rate climbs in proportion to the intensity of the exercise. When you are working as hard as you possibly can, your maximal heart rate is achieved. As you get older, that maximal heart rate decreases a little. When you work out at a steady intensity, your heart rate plateaus as it settles into the work that your muscles are doing. This is known as your steady state heart rate and can be used to estimate how fit you are. The lower your heart rate, the fitter you are.

During exercise, not only does your heart pump faster, but the amount of blood it pumps for every heartbeat also increases. This is called the **stroke volume**. The heart and body are clever at realising that you're working hard and the heart muscle starts squeezing more intensely. The heart pumps out the blood it receives back from the exercising muscles via the veins. As our muscles contract harder than usual, this pumps more blood back to the heart. Activation of nerves and hormones like adrenaline also make the muscle squeeze harder. It's an amazing process: the more blood the heart is given, the more it pumps out. And the amount of blood the heart pumps when we exercise can nearly double.

The way the heart increases the amount of blood it pumps is one of my favourite things about how it works. The heart is basically a muscular pump made up of millions of heart muscle cells. These cells contain highly specialised proteins called actin and myosin. They look a little like a rope being pulled along by many hands. When the muscle cell contracts, the myosin grabs onto the actin and pulls it towards itself, making the cell short and the whole muscle contract. Normally, only a few little myosin hands need to pull.

Imagine you are pulling on a rope with two of your friends – unfortunately there's only room for the three of you. There's only so much force you can generate with three people. Now imagine we stretch out the space that you're standing in and you can then add three more friends. Imagine how much harder you can pull!

When the extra blood returns to the heart, the muscle cells are stretched by the extra blood volume. This leaves much more room for the myosin hands to grab on to the actin rope and pull harder. This phenomenon is called the Frank–Starling mechanism, which explains that if we stretch the heart by adding volume, it will pump harder. Of course, there comes a point when the heart is too full and the myosin can't get its hands on the actin rope as they have been stretched or pushed too far away from it.

Just as squats strengthen your leg muscles, or bicep curls tone your arms, training your heart makes it a more effective pump. When you get fitter, a great deal is going on in your body. The skeletal muscles that move your joints work more effectively and they're able to exercise for longer. Your coordination and aptitude for the task improves so you feel less like a deer on ice. When it comes to your heart and lungs, endurance means that both develop the ability to deliver enough blood to the muscles for a longer period of time. With training, the heart is exactly like a well-oiled machine. It pumps better at rest and when you exercise, with stroke volume improving in all situations.

The heart of someone who has trained, say, for a half marathon slightly increases in size. If you're a runner, the hollow cavity of the heart gets bigger so more blood can be returned to it and more can be pumped out. If you're a weightlifter, the muscle grows bigger to overcome the jumps in blood pressure as you heave and puff to get those weights over your head. Exercise tells your body to continuously make more blood to improve fitness, and this lands back in the heart. Remember that the heart pumps out what it gets back.

When I was a third-year medical student, we had practical exams in which we performed physical examinations on volunteers, usually other university students. I examined a young man who removed his shirt to allow me to place my stethoscope on the front of his chest and listen to his heart. I counted a mere 35 beats in a minute and so I asked him if he worked out a lot. I guess he thought I was admiring his physique because he beamed with pride and said, 'Yeah, can you tell?'

I was actually referring to the fact that a resting heart rate of 35 is incredibly low and something usually only seen in particularly fit people. The heart becomes very efficient at pumping blood and so the body turns off all the nerve mechanisms that make the heart rate faster. Instead it turns on the parasympathetic nervous system that aims to 'rest and digest', slowing the heart rate and giving the heart longer to fill up.

All of these beneficial effects help to reduce our blood pressure too. The parasympathetic nervous system combined with direct effects on the blood vessels make them healthier and therefore they relax and dilate. The pressure inside them drops (which we measure by our blood pressure numbers) and this takes a load off the heart. Rather than pumping against pipes that are stiff and narrow, the heart doesn't need to work as hard. One of the things the heart hates the most is to pump against a high pressure, especially over a long term, such as when a person has high blood pressure.

Over time, blood pressure doesn't drop or change very much in people who are reasonably healthy or fit. However, if you are someone who has high blood pressure, this change in the tone or narrowness of blood vessels is crucially important. Blood pressure can drop with exercise by as much as 7 millimetres of mercury (mmHg, a measure of pressure) or more, which over time can help reduce high blood pressure.

When you've been training for a while, you may find that after you've been for a run or swim, instead of feeling like you might pass out, you feel good, or even great! You also recover faster. When you finish exercising, the heart rate stays up for a while to help the muscles recover, then drops back down to a resting heart rate. The fitter you are, the faster the heart rate returns to normal levels, generally speaking.

Exercise isn't all centred around the heart though. Your whole body joins in the fitness scene. Your muscles and other tissues open up or grow more capillaries. Capillaries are the tiniest of blood vessels and are the place where oxygen moves to the tissues that need it and waste is picked up for disposal. Having more capillaries means that your working muscles are more effectively able to get the oxygen they need to work harder.

The way the heart adapts and changes to these new situations is fascinating. Every day I can see these amazing changes in the flesh, so to speak. With the chest open and the heart on show, I can see how it looks when we give it more blood or take some away, or when we use medicine to make the heart pump faster or harder. When I watch this, I am in awe of how clever the heart is.

Cleverness is one thing, but exercise is probably one of the best medicines available. It is good for the heart, lungs, brain and bones, and can even reduce the risk of developing some types of cancer. When it comes to the heart, the gains from exercise are extraordinary and well worth the red face and sweatiness.

Paul's story

'This is Paul, he is 54 years old and he was pulled out of the pool while competing in the Australian Masters' swimming championships,' was how he was introduced to me. Without even asking, the look on his face said to us 'Why me?', pinpointing the unfairness of his situation. How did someone like Paul, who was fit and healthy, wind up in a hospital bed being examined by heart specialists?

A paragon of health, Paul had been in the middle of a race when the other competitors and spectators knew something was wrong. Midway up the lane he faltered, stopped and almost sank. The swimmers on either side pulled him to safety. Officials and competitors sprang into action, pressing on his chest and using an automated external defibrillator to deliver an electric shock and restore life. He was rushed to hospital, where a coronary angiogram showed that Paul had a very severe blockage in two of his coronary arteries. At the exact moment he started to sink to the bottom of the pool, Paul had suffered a heart attack and his heart had stopped beating.

Each day leading up to his surgery, Paul lamented the fact that he was slim, incredibly fit and had taken care of himself. He had never smoked and he rarely drank. He would look at us and ask if we saw many people like him. The answer was no. Most people who had lived like he had were rewarded with the healthiest of hearts. He was the last person we expected to need heart surgery. The fact of the matter was that somewhere along the line, Paul's genetics got the better of his lifestyle. We learnt that Paul's father had died suddenly when he was nearly 60 years old.

After his surgery, Paul had a different outlook. He was annoyed he hadn't even won a race for his troubles, which he would tell everyone who would listen with a cheeky grin. He had gone from asking 'Why me' to saying, 'Thank god it was then and there or else I might not be here'. Paul knew that without his physical fitness, he might not have survived. He also knew that his fitness enabled him to recover quickly after surgery. On his day of discharge, he assured me that he would soon be back in the pool, and that hopefully in his next race he'd walk away with a medal rather than a cut on his chest.

How exercise can save your life

The broader health benefits of exercise have been understood for thousands of years – after all, Hippocrates stated that 'walking is man's best medicine' around 400 BC. In modern times, a breakthrough study found that London bus drivers had more heart disease than their more active counterparts, bus conductors. It was the dawning of the realisation that exercise is vitally important for our hearts.

When we examine the rates of a certain disease in a particular group of people, we can correlate certain behaviours or risks and see who develops a disease and who doesn't. When looking at how exercise helps our hearts, it is interesting to look at the effects of doing the opposite. Sedentary behaviours or doing little exercise has been called 'the new smoking' in recent years. While that's not an entirely accurate description, it's a telling insight into the effect of exercise. When we reduce our sitting time to less than three hours a day, it's estimated that this can add nearly two years to our lives.

Other studies have looked directly at how much someone exerts themself when they exercise, using a measurement known as metabolic equivalents (METs). When a person can exercise at a higher capacity of METs, they drop their risk of heart disease in proportion to how hard they're working. Some studies report that exercise drops the risk of developing heart problems by as much as a third. This effect increases with the more exercise a person does in a day.

Epidemiology, which is the study of disease, its patterns and how it's changed by other factors (such as exercise, in this case), has provided us with plenty of evidence that 'exercise is good for you', but how exactly is exercise good for you and good for your heart?

Blood vessels are clever; they're a kind of organ in their own right. The inner lining of the blood vessels is called the endothelium and it has many functions other than providing a barrier. Most importantly, when the endothelium is healthy, our blood vessels are healthy. When our endothelium is sick or doesn't work well, our blood vessels get diseases like atheroma or develop plaque that blocks blood supply to our organs. If I had to choose one of my favourite parts of the body, the endothelium of the blood vessels would be my likely choice because of how smart it is.

When we exercise, the endothelium loves it. Blood pounds through the blood vessels and it causes extra stress along the endothelium. The clever endothelium reacts to that stress by creating a compound called nitric oxide, or NO. NO is incredibly important to the health of our blood vessels and when it's released, the blood vessels relax. This is valuable when we exercise because it allows more blood to get to our working muscles, but it's also important when we stop exercising.

The blood vessels' ability to regulate themselves and relax makes them healthier over time: they're not as thick and prone to forming plaque and they're more likely to relax easily, giving blood supply when it's needed and enabling the heart to pump against lower pressure. In the coronary arteries, the ability to relax in the short and long term allows the heart to get the blood it needs to exercise and operate well in daily life.

The benefits don't stop there. Exercise helps other parts of the body, including bone marrow, to activate various cells and hormones. These cells are known as endothelial progenitor cells. They are like the baby version of the cells making up the endothelium, which is mature and fully functional. We believe they help to heal damaged endothelium. When damaged, its function is impaired and it's more prone to developing plaque and blockages. For these reasons, exercise is beneficial for people who already have heart disease.

Aside from conditioning our heart and lungs to work more efficiently, exercise creates healthy blood vessels. The direct benefits of exercise to the heart and blood vessels are only half of the story though. All of our body's organs and processes are inextricably linked and the heart can be particularly vulnerable to ill health. Heart disease and heart attacks are often the end point of a number of diseases that make up the metabolic syndrome such as obesity, diabetes and high blood pressure. Exercise is able to improve the health of other tissues in the body, such as muscles and fat, which reduces the risk of diabetes, for example. This then places less stress on the heart.

Epidemiological studies have demonstrated the positive effects of being active on the development of diabetes and obesity. Being active significantly reduces the risk of developing diabetes, not only by reducing body weight but also by allowing insulin to work more effectively in the body. **Insulin** is an exceedingly important hormone. It's produced by a feather-shaped gland called the pancreas, which sits very close to the stomach. When our blood sugar rises, say after we eat, the pancreas releases insulin and our body grabs the sugars and fatty acids from the blood and stores it, usually in the form of fat or a glucose compound called glycogen. This is stored in the muscles so it's ready for use the next time we are active.

When we develop diabetes, or pre-diabetes, our muscles become ignorant to the signal from the insulin and don't take up the glucose and fatty acids. Rather than being stored away from the blood vessels, the glucose and fat stay in the bloodstream, causing injury and plaque formation. When our muscles contract, something amazing happens. The increased contraction causes the muscle cells to make more channels that can transport glucose from the blood into the muscles ready for use and away from the blood vessels where they can do damage. As a result, when diabetic patients exercise, their blood sugar levels often improve – a phenomenon known as improved insulin sensitivity. For people with diabetes, exercising as little as 150 minutes a week reduces their risk of dying and their reliance on medications.

As we have seen, weight loss is also a vitally important way to combat conditions such as diabetes and heart disease. Magazines and social media tout the benefits of exercise for weight loss but this effect goes beyond fitting into clothes you like. The best result you can gain from weight loss is to shift the fat that surrounds the organs, the visceral fat, which has a number of nasty effects on heart health. It makes and excretes hormones that promote diabetes, cause inflammation of the blood vessels and may even directly hurt your heart's ability to pump well. When you exercise, you not only see a shift in overall body weight, but studies have shown a specific loss of fat around the midsection. Waist circumference is a surrogate marker for the dangerous fat that lives beneath the surface, around and in the organs.

What about patients who already have heart disease? This group should exercise more than anyone. Cardiac rehabilitation is an exercise program prescribed to people with heart conditions and those who have had a heart attack or heart surgery. It is largely a graded program, supervised by exercise physiologists and physiotherapists. This kind of exercise improves symptoms and even quality of life and chances of survival. Patients on this program tend to recover much faster. Even more useful is having a baseline level of fitness that allows us to approach any illness with a real chance of recovering well.

Exercise is also great for many other things that feed into our heart health, like our sleep, our mood and alleviating depression. All of these things, when not in balance, place a great deal of unnecessary stress on the heart. Exercise is a medicine that is wonderful for our whole bodies, particularly our hearts.

How much exercise?

Many years ago, after a heart attack or major surgery, patients would be prescribed bed rest. This advice goes back to the late 1700s when, after a heart attack, doctors told patients to stay in bed for six weeks for fear of stressing the sick heart. Instead of recovering, however, patients often developed an array of complications and lost vital muscle mass and fitness as a result. Much of the knowledge we have gained about the terrible effects of being immobilised for long periods of time has come from the space race. In space, astronauts are essentially immobilised and they develop a number of conditions, such as muscle wasting, causing multiple illnesses when they return to gravity.

In the 1940s 'chair therapy' was prescribed for recovery from a heart attack, which is exactly as it sounds: you sat in a chair for six long weeks. Over the years, medical science changed its views on rehabilitation, to the point where now I give my patients instructions to walk daily and then walk some more. Most patients do laps of the ward and eventually laps of their house and street. Occasionally someone asks for a different exercise prescription. I've been asked about everything from horseriding to sex as appropriate exercise after heart surgery. I always recommend walking because it's easy, cheap and achievable.

What about those of us who are healthy: what is the right amount of exercise? If we consider exercise a medicine (and a good one at that), we need a prescription. We need to determine which type of exercise we should do, for how long and how hard we need to work to get a benefit. There is so much conflicting information around, with claims abounding about which exercise is the best: this one is a miracle cure, that one will burn the most calories and another will give you arms to rival Michelle Obama. If we put calories and the former US First Lady aside, what does science say we should be doing?

When the World Health Organisation identifies a health issue as important, it speaks volumes. The WHO has identified daily activity targets for all age groups: children, adults and the elderly. For adults aged 18 to 64, the minimum target is 150 minutes per week of moderate-intensity aerobic activity or 75 minutes of vigorous-intensity activity. That's, say, walking when you can hold a conversation versus running when, if someone asked you to talk, you wouldn't even have the spare breath to laugh at the suggestion.

That's just the baseline. To add to those benefits, the WHO suggests 300 minutes of moderate or 150 minutes of vigorous activity per week, plus muscle strengthening two or more days a week. It seems like a lot, doesn't it? But the WHO isn't endorsing 300 long minutes on a treadmill or anything so strict. Physical activity isn't just hitting a gym or running kilometres on end. It's everything we do that is physical: from our exercise of choice, to walking to work or around the office, playing games or doing housework. Yes, the world's premier health organisation considers sweeping the floors a contribution to your health.

If you do the bare minimum, it's essentially two and a half hours of exercise weekly. Many of us might think we would struggle to find that time. I know some days or weeks, I certainly do. We are all incredibly busy. I try to exercise before work, which means getting up and being out the door before 5.15 in the morning to fit my exercise in. My evenings are too unpredictable or I'm too tired after a day at work to want to exercise. I know I'm not alone here: we work, parent, socialise, sleep, volunteer or undertake any number of other commitments that make us time poor and make us feel as though we're too exhausted to exercise.

The magic number of 150 minutes a week or 30 minutes a day came from a large study of more than 50,000 people in the United States. The study found that even a slow jog resulted in an increase in life expectancy of up to three years. The study compared people who ran or jogged with those who were more sedentary. It is unclear though how much of that benefit comes from just running. As you'd expect, the people who were runners were much more motivated to be healthier overall so they didn't smoke, have diabetes or high blood pressure. That's not to say that the information gained from this study wasn't useful. Scientific studies are often contending with information that might muddy the water, a factor we call 'confounding'. The information from studies like this can be analysed to control for, or remove, the effects of these confounders. However, there is no denying that if you are already healthy, you're more likely to exercise and that becomes a kind of self-fulfilling prophecy.

What kind of exercise?

Many quality studies have shown that when it comes to exercise intensity, more is more. The higher-intensity exercisers tend to get a much higher benefit from their workouts. The classic comparison is running versus walking. Running has been shown to have at least double the benefit of walking when it comes to reducing the risk of dying from heart disease, and in less time too. A five-minute run is equivalent to a 15-minute walk.

Running is tough, though, especially when you first start, and some research has shown that even for less serious runners, injury is common. Given this, reducing running time to between five and fifteen minutes a day might mean you lessen the likelihood of injuries, while still gaining some of the heart benefits. Running may give you more bang for your buck, but at the end of the day, if you hate it you won't do it. Walking may get you there slower but it does have some distinct advantages over running: it's quite a social endeavour (walking and talking is a great way to catch up with friends and work out) and is less likely to result in injury.

When I consider this research, I find it easy to be overcome with guilt. I can't run like I used to, after a knee injury, and sometimes I just don't enjoy it. Am I doing myself a disservice by not choosing the most effective exercise possible? Absolutely not. Solely on a numbers basis the science is very much in favour of running, but it has to translate to the real world that we live in. So if you can't run or you can't stand running, and walking with your friends or with the dogs is what you want to do, then that is absolutely fine. Remember that the benefit from exercise largely comes from just doing it, not being an elite athlete. In fact, any movement at all is to be encouraged.

What about other types of exercise? High-intensity interval training (HIIT) has been popularised lately as a workout that gives you maximal outcome from a short, sharp workout. The idea behind HIIT is that you work in intervals, doing some sort of aerobic exercise at such an intensity that it can only be done for short bursts. It's popular, but is it better? Better is a strong word when it comes to the science of exercise, because it studies real life, which is messy. That being said, a number of studies have shown that HIIT is great for reducing blood pressure, improving levels of high-density cholesterol (good cholesterol), decreasing blood glucose and improving how sensitive our fat and muscles are to insulin.

Yoga is another form of exercise that is gaining popularity in the West, with its emphasis on the body as well as the mind. Yoga reduces all of the risks for heart disease. It improves body weight, good cholesterol (HDL) and blood pressure, although it isn't great at reducing blood sugar levels. Yoga compares very favourably with other forms of exercise though. In fact, some cardiac rehabilitation programs have started using yoga to help patients recover from their heart attacks.

There are so many ways to be active. You can dance, you can run, cycle or swim. The fact remains that being active is undeniably the best thing you can do for yourself. How much is too little, how much is too much? The basic idea is to get moving: just do something. Even if running is 'better' in some regards, simply finding what you enjoy and what you can commit to will bring huge benefits. In reality, what most of us need is just to start exercising. My rule of thumb? Some is better than none and more is better than some.

chapter 8
RED WINE, DARK CHOCOLATE AND SUPERFOODS

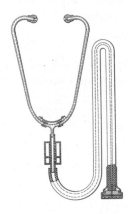

Wine is constant proof that God loves us and loves to see us happy

BENJAMIN FRANKLIN, SCIENTIST AND POLITICIAN

There are some incredibly sad aspects of my job. I met a man one day who had had what we call 'palliative' surgery for a particularly nasty form of lung-related cancer called mesothelioma. It's cancer of the lining of the chest and is strongly linked to asbestos. What's terrible about this type of cancer is its dreadful prognosis. My family knows this first-hand – it was the kind of cancer that my grandfather died of. This poor man had probably been exposed to asbestos when he was building his house. He had an operation to try to control some of his symptoms and enable him to live more comfortably for as long as possible.

He came to hospital because his breathing had worsened. I sat down with him in the emergency department to talk about what had been going wrong. He was upset that what little independence he had left was being destroyed by the progression of his disease. I remember feeling an intense sense of frustration that medicine had not yet been able to provide a cure for this dreadful disease. Through his tears, he told me that not even the juice had worked. What juice was that? I asked. In the hope of finding a cure, he had sought counsel from his local health food store and been assured that their special supplements and carrot juices would lengthen his life. He bawled into his hands thinking about the $300 a week the futile carrot juice was costing him, which was money he could not afford to spend.

If faced with a terminal illness, I don't think any of us can say for sure that we wouldn't try anything available to us. This man had put his faith in the promise of healing superfoods and supplements and, as he described it, the only thing it was doing was 'making him poor'. The disease eventually took hold and he passed away. Part of me wanted to visit that health store and berate them for taking advantage of a dying man. Part of me was sympathetic, wondering what superfoods I would try if my life was in the balance.

I recently discovered that when it comes to my own health, so-called superfoods have lodged themselves in my subconscious, as they have for many people. I am unlucky enough to have a strong family history of high blood pressure and heart disease, so I had finally decided to pull my head out of the sand and get my heart checked by my doctor. As the cuff tightened, it wasn't good news. My genes, my stress and my recent lapse in exercise had betrayed me and I had blood pressure that was much too high. It was a wake-up call, so I marched myself down to the supermarket to add lots of fresh fruit and vegetables to the pantry.

As I walked through the supermarket, I wondered where the superfoods for high blood pressure were, making a mental note to get a bottle of red wine because it's 'good for the heart'. What an odd thought. Why did I think superfoods and red wine would be my saviours?

The idea of food as medicine is gaining momentum as we realise the impact of what we eat on fighting or feeding disease. Is a glass of red wine a day really going to make your heart healthy? Is dark chocolate as good for you as you may try to justify? Many of us are interested in the latest iterations of the red wine debate or learning what the latest superfood is. It's hard not to buy into the promise of the newest health food saviour.

The funny thing is that before I started my own search for superfoods in the supermarket aisles, I had thought the buzz around certain foods was interesting, but could not believe that they were the cure-all they were often purported to be. However, I had never gone sifting through the evidence to see what science said about them.

Red wine

How many times have you clinked glasses of wine and felt virtuous because you were drinking red? Red wine often features in the media as something that you should drink for your health, particularly for your heart. In general, alcohol consumption, especially to excess, is something we are told to avoid for the sake of our bodies.

Red wine and other alcohol are two very different beasts. Alcohol, in beer, white wine or spirits, doesn't have many health benefits, especially when you have 'too much'. Current guidelines tell us that we should have no more than two standard drinks per day and no more than four in one sitting. A standard drink is a lot smaller than we might think, so for many people, exceeding this benchmark is easier than it sounds.

Studies over many years have demonstrated that while a glass of wine after work or a beer at a summer barbecue might be a great pleasure, alcohol is not great for us. It tends to cause problems in a dose-related effect: so, the more you have, the more problems it causes. The list of diseases that arise from drinking too much alcohol is extraordinarily long, including liver disease and some cancers. Countless studies have looked at how much a person drinks and compared that to their risk of heart disease. Most of the time, what we see is that the people who drink the most, as well as those who drink nothing at all, have the highest risk of heart disease. The so-called 'moderate' drinkers seem to be the best protected.

These studies have a couple of flaws. Firstly, asking people to report how much they drink is not always reliable. People often think that they should drink less, so they say that they drink less than they actually do. Recently, an interesting explanation was offered as to why non-drinkers fared worse than moderate drinkers. Among people who drank no alcohol whatsoever, some studies discovered that teetotallers were more likely to have previously been heavier drinkers. Which means they might have already exposed themselves to the risks associated with heavy drinking.

Giving up drinking is great, but what this illustrates is that life is more than a snapshot. Our lifestyle and health matters over longer periods, not just right now. That includes not having periods of excess in between the times when our drinking is restrained. More finessed studies, not just observational ones, have suggested that for all of us, reducing the amount of alcohol we consume is a great idea. However, there is an unexpected finding that still persists: small amounts of alcohol may actually protect our hearts.

Researchers believe that alcohol may change the levels of HDL, or good cholesterol, depending on how much we drink. High blood pressure and alcohol consumption often go together. However, at lower levels of consumption, alcohol may relax blood vessels and so lower blood pressure. It's not entirely clear what mechanisms might be at play; this is still coming to light. One interesting possibility relates to an enzyme called alcohol dehydrogenase that is slightly different in each of us. Some of us have a small variation in this enzyme that slows down how alcohol is processed and disposed of by our bodies. It also may encourage the liver to make more HDL cholesterol, which is thought to be protective.

Alcohol use is also associated with an abnormal heart rhythm called atrial fibrillation, which is the most common type of heart rhythm problem. For each drink we have per day, our risk of atrial fibrillation increases. This is probably due to the fact that alcohol depresses the pumping ability of the heart and might directly cause problems to the heart's electrical systems.

So why is red wine different? Here's an even better question: *is* red wine any different?

Just to be clear: in excess, red wine is the same kind of bad as a few too many beers a night. It's not the alcohol in red wine that has the benefits, it is all the other gear. The idea that red wine might be protective is sometimes called the 'French Paradox'. In the late 1970s a researcher noted that, despite a relatively high-fat diet filled with cheese and butter, the French had one of the lowest rates of death from heart attacks. Another finding showed that in regions of France where people preferred a white with dinner to a red, there were worse survival rates from heart attacks.

This *petit observation intéressant* led researchers to investigate why red wine might be powerful enough to take on butter. Around the same time as the French Paradox was noted, the war on fat was gaining momentum. It seemed remarkable that red wine might be potent enough to negate all the problems caused by public enemy number one.

Around 20 years later, experiments showed that even small amounts of red wine contained a substance called phenol. Phenols are a type of antioxidant and there is one that is specifically in red wine called resveratrol. Resveratrol runs around our blood vessels mopping up free radicals. Free radicals are little angry molecules of oxygen that we all produce as side effects of the normal cellular metabolic processes in our bodies. They are harmful to our tissues and so our body has free radicals scavenged by antioxidants. Some antioxidants we make, some we get in our diet. Back to France, where using wine in cooking is common and meat is often marinated in red wine, the result is that antioxidants knock out free radicals in the meat before it is even eaten.

Resveratrol is good at preventing the oxidisation of LDL, or bad cholesterol. When LDL is oxidised, an oxygen molecule is added to it. This is like arming that molecule to go out and cause carnage. An oxidised molecule of LDL is much more easily retained in the blood vessel walls, which is where plaque can form. If red wine can prevent that LDL from getting angry and activated, it may lose some of its disease-causing ability.

That's not the only way in which red wine can be useful. Resveratrol is also able to induce the endothelium (lining of our blood vessels) to make nitric oxide. We've met nitric oxide before: it's a potent vasodilator. That is, it causes blood vessels to relax. Red wine helps our bodies make nitric oxide, which means that there is a wide-open flow to our hearts and all other organs of beautiful, nutrient-rich blood. Red wine and indeed alcohol in general may be useful at keeping the blood thin, by calming down the clotting process when it's not needed. If you can imagine how much better it is to push thinner rather than thicker blood through a tube, you get the idea of why that can be useful. It's all about good flow when it comes to blood supply, and some scientists believe red wine may deliver this in spades.

It is believed there may be a number of other beneficial mechanisms activated in red wine. Red wine may help to keep the heart muscle supple by blocking scarring in the heart, or blocking enzymes called angiotensin-II that indirectly increase blood pressure. This is incidentally also a target of very important and commonly used medications called ACE inhibitors. ACE inhibitors are used to lower blood pressure and help people with heart failure. What's fascinating is that the benefits of red wine are still gained when the wine has the alcohol removed. It's mostly about the grape that is used to make red wine.

Research on the effects of red wine on heart disease is a work in progress. An exciting possibility is that the specific substances in red wine could be turned into a medication that treats or prevents heart disease. New information, however, can be at times in conflict with previous research on red wine, alcohol and heart disease. For the time being, studies show that red wine has some great potential benefits for our hearts, but only if we consume it sparingly. The same goes for alcohol. At low doses, alcohol is enjoyable and probably good for us. At higher doses, alcohol is bad news. Don't drink to be healthy, rather drink (judiciously) because you are.

Dark chocolate

Certain to make the news and be discussed repeatedly is any scientific study that finds chocolate is good for us. Any quasi-scientific whisper that chocolate might be healthy is like a free pass to go crazy on a whole block of it.

The distinction between dark chocolate and the sweeter (and possibly less healthy) milk chocolate is incredibly important. It was for one of my patients. At 52 she lived a relatively normal life, working as a paralegal in a busy law firm, and was on her feet all day. Three years earlier, she had been diagnosed with diabetes after complaining to her GP that she was constantly tired. Diabetes tends to hide away for a period of time before it's diagnosed, and in that time it can do a lot of damage. Which, in this patient's case, it had.

The diabetes and high blood sugars had attacked blood vessels in her legs, eyes and heart. At an age that by today's standards was not very old, she was facing open-heart surgery.

I sat on her bed as she looked me square in the eyes and said, 'This is all my fault. I don't check my blood sugar, I eat chocolate every day and I never deny myself anything.' I was a little shocked, because few people are so blunt when it comes to admitting the ways in which they don't look after themselves. And she took the same blunt approach in responding to her illness by 'pulling her head in', a great Australian colloquialism for addressing your shortcomings and fixing the problem. On a ward round a few days after her surgery, she proudly showed me how she had switched from her favourite sweet and milky chocolate to dark chocolate.

Chocolate, for all the positive publicity it receives, probably doesn't have the same beneficial effects on our health as fruit and vegetables. That doesn't mean that there is nothing beneficial there though. A little like red wine, dark chocolate is rich in antioxidants. An antioxidant group called flavonoids are thought to be the heroes here. Flavonoids are antioxidants that are found in plants and, just like the antioxidants found in wine, they scavenge up any harmful free radicals, preventing them from doing damage to our cells.

Chocolate is made from a plant. Cocoa beans produced by the cacao tree are ground, roasted and formed into a paste and added to milk and sweeteners or other flavours. These plant origins mean that chocolate contains all those lovely plant-based antioxidants. Similarly to when we drink red wine, when we eat chocolate free radicals are mopped up and the endothelium produces nitric oxide, causing blood vessels to relax and blood to flow smoothly. It probably also improves the ratio of good cholesterol to bad cholesterol in the blood and helps our bodies respond much more effectively to insulin.

In theory, chocolate has the hallmarks of a heart-health crusader. Many epidemiological or observational studies have looked at how our hearts benefit from chocolate. A large recent study showed that in men and women who ate up to 100 grams of chocolate a day, the risk of heart disease was much lower. To put that in perspective, a single square of chocolate is around 8 grams. Chocolate eaters were also less likely to die from a heart attack. Interestingly, the findings weren't able to show a difference between dark and other types of chocolate. That being said, this was a pretty weak finding of the study and most other science suggests that dark chocolate has the race won when it comes to heart disease.

Another interesting study used human blood vessel cells, taken from umbilical cords and grown in a lab, and almost bathed them in chocolate. The lab isolated the good parts of the chocolate, specifically the antioxidant flavonoids, and incubated the blood vessel cells in them to prove that the flavonoids found in dark chocolate were great at making healthy blood vessels. That data was used to show that in people with blood vessel disease, such as peripheral arterial disease, eating dark chocolate made their blood vessels perform much better. The vessels relaxed and blood could get more easily to where it needed to be, meaning that these patients could walk again as blood made it to their hungry working muscles. People who have blockages of the blood vessels in their legs often can't walk far; their muscles are starved of the oxygen they need. It was thought that the dark chocolate helped them recover, in a sense. It's a similar situation in the heart. Working out ways to improve blood supply to the heart is vitally important for healthy hearts.

We've come across inflammation several times now. Just to recap: inflammation is the body's attempt at fighting things it thinks aren't good for it. When it goes a little harder than it should, inflammation can cause damage. In our hearts and blood vessels, unchecked inflammation starts cascades of processes that harm the vessels and the heart. Being able to keep inflammation in check is very important. Cocoa and the flavonoids contained in it are quite good at stopping the cells from producing inflammatory hormone-like molecules called cytokines. It's this action that may also stop the development of irregular heart rhythms, such as atrial fibrillation, in chocolate eaters.

Dark chocolate and milk chocolate share a lot of the same compounds, such as flavonoids. Dark chocolate, though, has a few advantages over milk chocolate. Firstly, it contains higher concentrations of antioxidants. Secondly, it also has less of the stuff that might undo all the antioxidants' good work, such as saturated fat and sugar.

A little like red wine, we aren't about to start taking out our prescription pads and prescribing dark chocolate just yet. Nor does gorging ourselves on dark chocolate mean that we get a free pass from doing all the other things we should for our hearts, like exercising and eating fruit and vegetables. If you must have chocolate, it is probably best to stick with darker chocolate of at least 70 per cent cocoa to get the health benefits along with the treat.

Coffee and tea

I have two observations to make about coffee. The first is that it smells awful to me. As someone who drinks neither coffee nor tea, I know that puts me in the minority because most coffee drinkers I know love it! The second is that everyone around me seems to drink coffee. Common sayings like 'First, coffee' are an ode to how people can't get going in the morning without their habitual eye-opener. Despite this, I can't bring myself to be a coffee drinker; it is a taste that I never became accustomed to. Very occasionally I almost regret this because a news article tells me that drinking coffee or tea is actually 'good for you'.

In the United States around 80 per cent of people drink coffee; nearly 60 per cent of adults drink it daily. Coffee culture is a modern phenomenon in Australia, with people being very specific about what kind of coffee they drink. Even tea is having a moment, with whole stores dedicated to selling more types of tea than you ever thought possible. It becomes a habit, a taste and an experience.

A little like chocolate, when a study is published about the supposed health benefits of coffee, the internet goes wild, with people viewing it as permission to indulge their favourite vice. However, many studies over the years have been conflicting when it comes to the health benefits of coffee. Some studies have shown that people who drink a lot of coffee may have a higher risk of heart disease. This association was strongest for people under the age of 55 who drank more than four cups a day. In comparison, a number of other big studies have showed a decline in heart disease for coffee drinkers. It's possible that studies that found coffee drinking wasn't great for us may have been subject to confounders, such as the way people took their coffee.

Compounds in coffee have a number of effects on the heart and blood vessels. In addition to caffeine, coffee contains phenolic acids and potassium. There isn't a consensus on how coffee may be good for us, but it's thought to be beneficial in reducing inflammation and the body's sensitivity to insulin. This may be very good for the heart and blood vessels as it can minimise the number of damaging substances they're exposed to.

Coffee can directly oppose the action of hormones that relax blood vessels and so can slightly increase blood pressure. It also enhances the actions of the sympathetic nervous system on the heart, causing the heart to beat faster. That's the thumping in your chest when you have an extra coffee. Interestingly, if you have a cup of coffee (or more) every day, your body gets used to these reactions and is able to ignore these potentially troublesome effects. For example, regular coffee drinkers don't get the same spike in blood pressure that less habitual coffee drinkers get when they have a coffee.

When it comes to drinking coffee for health, the truth probably lies in a grey area. When all these studies are considered, the overall trend is that drinking some coffee is not bad for your heart. It's probably even a little beneficial for your heart. But not as healthy as exercise or a balanced diet.

The other important thing to keep in mind is how you have your coffee: adding sugar is not good. When looking at coffee drinkers who have had heart attacks, these people tended to add a lot of sugar to their diet in general, as well as to their coffee. So, for health, coffee is probably fine, and may even be good for your heart. However, skip the sugar and get your caffeine hit *au naturel*.

Superfoods

I am perpetually overwhelmed by reports detailing the latest superfood. With headlines like 'Five superfoods that Jesus ate', it's a battle not to click on the link and get drawn into the news of some unaffordable exotic berry or unpronounceable grain. With promises of longevity and health, superfoods seem to be the cure to our growing personal and societal epidemic of ill health. I try to look at these claims with a healthy dose of scepticism and scientific curiosity, but as I admitted earlier, I reflexively found myself thinking of superfoods as a way to deal with my own hypertension.

'Superfood' is more of a marketing term than a scientific one. Generally, the label is given to foods that have a high nutritional benefit. In fact, when a food is labelled as a superfood in the media, sales of that food spike significantly. Consumption of these superfoods is disproportionately higher in people with higher incomes. This is hardly surprising given that these foods are often relatively expensive.

Foods that are often called superfoods include easily attainable staples like broccoli and blueberries as well as the slightly more exotic goji berries, spelt grains, quinoa and kale. They are generally foods that are high in vitamins, minerals and antioxidants, just like red wine and dark chocolate. And, just like red wine, these plant-based foods produce antioxidants called phenols, of which resveratrol is one, and basically keep our blood vessels healthy by mopping up free radicals and producing nitric oxide.

In a number of superfoods, the active ingredients that form the basis of their super-status are actually found more abundantly elsewhere. Kale is constantly labelled a superfood, but Brussels sprouts and other green leafy vegetables are just as healthy. Rocket has more nitrates, which lower blood pressure, than beetroot. Salmon has nearly double the good omega-3 fatty acids, which are important for maintenance of a healthy fat profile in blood, than chia seeds. All are much cheaper and easier to come by.

In theory, so-called superfoods are good for us. They tend to be fruits and vegetables or grains that are low in sugar and fat and high in micronutrients. Here's the question though: are superfoods any better for us than boring old vegetables that are cheaper and much easier to get our hands on? The crux of the matter is this: no single food, super or otherwise, can make up for an otherwise ordinary diet. In fact, European legislation says that no food can be called, marketed or claimed as a superfood unless you can prove its health benefits. The ban has been in place since 2007, which was incredibly forward thinking.

The testing of superfoods isn't carried out in a way that is necessarily applicable to daily life. Compounds in superfoods that are good for us are often isolated in a lab and then given to cells to see how they respond. Those results are then extrapolated to the population. That is, we see a good thing in a test tube so we think that it might be good in real life, too. But we don't know for sure. Unlike general fruit and vegetable consumption or even red wine and chocolate consumption, there aren't enough people eating these superfoods to enable us to study how healthy they are or how many heart attacks they have had, and how this might relate to their superfood diet. So, we can't say that a superfood is a true panacea.

When it comes to superfoods, the science isn't there. Superfoods cannot compensate for obesity, inactivity or simply having an unlucky combination of genes. Are they harmful? Probably not. Should you pay more for them? If you like them and are willing to spend more on your grocery bill, go for it. I love quinoa for its flavour as well as its benefits as a whole grain, not because it is a superfood.

The science behind superfoods may change over time and if there is a food that is going to help us lose weight, reduce heart attacks or live longer then that is excellent. For now, however, you do not have to consume superfoods to be truly healthy. Healthy foods are available everywhere and are generally much cheaper. Foods like salmon, everyday fruit and vegetables and standard whole grains are backed by science as helping improve the health of your heart by lowering blood pressure, reducing bad cholesterol, cultivating a healthy gut microbiome and keeping a healthy weight.

chapter 9
DEPRESSION: CAN A HEART BE BLUE?

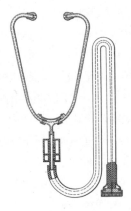

Mental pain is less dramatic than physical pain, but it is more common and also more hard to bear. The frequent attempt to conceal mental pain increases the burden: it is easier to say 'My tooth is aching' than to say 'My heart is broken'
C.S. LEWIS, WRITER, ACADEMIC AND THEOLOGIAN

I sat in my clinic, ready to see my last patient for the day. He had come for his check-up, six weeks after his heart surgery. I remembered him of course, but it was not an intense, crisp memory. To me, this usually means that surgery has gone well, the patient has recovered easily and returned home. Not remembering specific dramatic details usually means that there were none, which in heart surgery is probably a good thing. I looked through his paperwork and refreshed my memory of his medical issues, noticing that he was a very heavy smoker and had trouble quitting. I made a mental note to see how that was going.

It turned out I didn't need the mental note. He sat down in my room and the smell of cigarette smoke in the air was thick. I knew that my room would have the distinct odour of smoke for the rest of the day. I asked him how he was going, looked at his wounds and his chest X-ray. Everything looked good. We went through his medications and then he dropped a comment into the conversation that piqued my interest. 'I've been hanging out for this appointment. All I do is sit at home and do nothing.'

I asked him what he meant by 'hanging out for this appointment', and the floodgates opened. He told me that he had had two relationship breakdowns before he was admitted to hospital with a heart attack followed by heart surgery. During his hospital stay his partner had left him, but he had to face the indignity of going back to their shared home after discharge until he could find somewhere else to live. This wasn't easy because he couldn't work and so was on a pension that barely covered the cost of rent and food. He had no friends and no family, so he sat at home all day. The only highlights were going to physiotherapy and doctors' visits. My heart was pained to think that coming to see me, someone he really didn't know, could pass as a highlight.

I asked, 'Do you think you're depressed?' and he replied, 'Of course I am, what with everything that is going on. It's why I can't give up smoking: what else do I have to do with my time?'

My brief consult turned into a much longer one for two reasons. Firstly, I was so sad for this man who thought that this hospital visit, among the cold, clinical rooms and corridors, was something to look forward to. Secondly, I wanted to sort out his mental state, not just as a person but as a doctor. Depression is a horrible condition to live with; more and more we are learning just how bad depression is for the body. Particularly for the heart. I'm not a psychiatrist but I wanted this man to get better, mind and body, and both needed to be in good working order for that to happen.

A brief recap of depression

We talk about depression much more than we used to. Which is a good thing. Around the world, more than 300 million people are affected by depression. In Australia, around 1 million people have depression, around one in 20, and over their lifetime nearly half of Australians will have a mental disorder. Those statistics are similar around the world, with 6.7 per cent of Americans being depressed, and around one in four to one in six in the United Kingdom.

Depression is far worse than just being a little sad, and if we keep that in mind, we can see why depression might affect our hearts. People with depression have a really low mood that lasts beyond a couple of weeks. Depression also causes something called anhedonia, which means that sufferers lose pleasure from things that used to give them pleasure. It's also associated with feelings of worthlessness, guilt and sometimes anxiety. This syndrome also impacts our bodies physically, causing changes in appetite, energy levels and sleep.

Depression can be triggered by a traumatic life event, like having a heart problem, for example. But this isn't the only factor that can precipitate depression. Our genes are an important influence, with some estimates putting 30 per cent of the risk squarely on what we inherit from our parents. The remaining 70 per cent is from our environment, including our personality, coping style and age, and can also be affected by long-term stress or a major life-changing event. It's important to know that depression is an illness, just like heart disease, that is rooted in biochemical changes in the brain. It does not mean that you can't cope. Just as you would see a doctor for a broken bone, seeing a doctor for depression is no different.

It may seem odd for a heart surgeon to be writing about depression. The brain is a long way from the heart, right? The fact is though, the brain and the heart are much more connected and dependent on each other than we previously knew.

We are starting to appreciate the stress that depression places on our bodies and especially our hearts. Years ago, having a low mood after a heart attack may have been met with a pat on the back and a brief (yet hopefully well-meaning) instruction to 'keep your chin up'. Nowadays, depression is recognised as a serious risk for not only developing heart disease, but also for impairing the ability to recover and stay well. In fact, patients are at risk after suffering a number of physical diseases, not to mention after serious illness as well. It becomes a nasty cycle. But how exactly does the head hurt the heart? Or can it be the other way around? Does having heart disease make you depressed?

Chicken or egg?

Being seriously ill can bring on depression. It's a common finding in a number of patients who have a sudden medical problem. At the same time, depression is, as we've said, now recognised as a risk factor for a number of illnesses, and heart disease is one of them. It's a little like the chicken and egg conundrum. Is my heart sick because I'm depressed or am I depressed because I have a sick heart?

If we were to look at all of the people who have heart disease, including 'stable' heart disease, the rates of depression are reported at around 31 to 45 per cent. People who have heart disease such as angina or have had a heart attack are three times as likely to suffer depression as the general population. Hearts aren't alone in this: cancer patients have around the same levels of depression. It makes perfect sense that a life-threatening or life-changing disease would impact your mental health.

In a study of more than 93,000 women, people who had depression were more likely to have heart troubles – almost 1.5 times that seen in people who didn't have depression. Interestingly, depression has been shown to be a risk factor for a heart attack even without traditional risks like high blood pressure or diabetes being present. In otherwise physically healthy people, depression can be enough to cause damage to the heart and blood vessels. One study even showed that having depression increased the risk of a heart attack by 1.6 times.

If this and other risk factors converge, depression is incredibly bad for you and your heart. This is when the numbers really start getting scary. Patients who have had a heart attack and have depression are nearly 2.5 times more likely to have another heart attack or die from their heart disease. These people are also more likely to be readmitted to hospital with heart problems. It doesn't matter if they had depression before their heart attack or if they developed it after, either situation is not good. However, if the heart attack brings on the depression, this is the group that struggles the most with their heart health.

How does the heavy fog of depression cause difficulties all the way down in our hearts? Once again, inflammation is at play. Depression may seem tucked away in the brain, but it causes many different cells in the body to release substances that are a kind of hormone called cytokines. These pro-inflammatory cytokines activate the immune system. This can possibly perpetuate depression but the ill effects also spill over into the rest of the body. People who are depressed often experience crushing fatigue, which is linked to these cytokines and the widespread inflammation they cause.

In order to scientifically prove that depression and the inflammation associated with it caused heart issues, cytokines linked to depression were measured in the bloodstreams of people with the disease. The cytokines were studied to see if they caused trouble in the hearts and blood vessels. And this was exactly what was seen. The same cytokine levels that are heightened in depression are thought to directly injure the heart and cause blood vessels to clog up.

Even without the inflammation caused by depression, there are still plenty of people with depression getting heart disease. This tells us that there is more than one factor at play when it comes to linking depression and heart disease.

Depression affects our blood vessels, which can also make our hearts sick. Partly due to inflammation and other factors that are still unclear, the endothelium (lining of the blood vessels) doesn't work as well as it should when a patient is depressed. A healthy endothelium, as we know, is important to prevent artery-clogging plaque from forming. The endothelium normally produces and reacts to nitric oxide, which causes blood vessels to relax and lets blood flow easily through them. In patients who have depression, the blood vessels aren't as good at relaxing, even in response to nitric oxide. This not only impairs the flow of blood, but it can also make the vessel prone to injury. An injured blood vessel is highly prone to forming plaque and it can't give the tissues and organs the blood supply they need.

You may have already heard that aspirin has made huge dents in the rates of heart attacks, and it's routinely given to people having a heart attack. Aspirin's life-saving properties come from its ability to stop blood from clotting inside diseased arteries. It does this by stopping tiny blood cells called platelets from clumping together and lodging on particularly nasty plaque in the heart's coronary arteries, which causes a heart attack. Just like virtually every cell and organ in the body, platelets are influenced by hormones. And an important hormone in platelet function is serotonin. This may be ringing bells for you because depression and serotonin are often spoken of together, mainly because serotonin's other job is in the brain. Serotonin is a neurotransmitter, which is a kind of molecule that signals between neurons and parts of the brain and is strongly implicated in depression.

One of my favourite things about the body and science is the way everything is interconnected. In the bodies of people with depression and particularly in the brain, a chemical transmitter called serotonin is thought to be low, leading to the major symptoms of depression. When we give people with depression a drug called selective serotonin reuptake inhibitor (SSRI), we see the levels of serotonin shooting around the brain rise and people feel better.

But we also see an interesting effect on platelets. When serotonin is taken up into platelets, they clump together to start making blood clots. Possibly due to low serotonin, depressed patients may have hyperactive platelets that travel around the body, looking for vessels to stick to and clog up. The SSRI drugs inhibit serotonin being snuck back inside platelets. The lack of serotonin inside the platelets means they aren't as good at sticking together and therefore the blood becomes much stickier. Treating depression may have the side effect of treating the abnormal blood clotting that causes heart attacks.

That is not the whole story. One of the ways the brain communicates with the body is by the use of hormones. Hormones can reach further than the brain and nerves sometimes can. This is called a neurohormonal mechanism, which is exactly as it sounds: brain or nerves and hormones.

In patients with heart problems, we see increased levels of adrenaline and its cousin, noradrenaline. They can make the heart pump faster and harder and need more oxygen, and increase blood pressure. These are useful mechanisms if you are running from danger, but not if you have a sick heart. In patients with heart failure, high blood levels of these hormones can mean their chances of survival are lowered. One medicine used for heart failure called a beta-blocker has a role in directly opposing the storm of unnecessary work that adrenaline and noradrenaline can cause.

Patients with depression appear to have an imbalance between the two neural systems that excrete these hormones. The sympathetic nervous system is our fight-or-flight system. It's also responsible for pumping out adrenaline and noradrenaline. The opposing system is the parasympathetic nervous system, responsible for our body's ability to 'rest and digest'. Patients with depression tend to have an imbalance between the two systems, with the sympathetic nervous system being far too in control.

In patients with depression, this causes a phenomenon called reduced heart-rate variability. Heart-rate variability is the variation between each heartbeat and, when that variability is reduced, it is a marker of a heart that gets too much 'fight or flight' and not enough 'rest and digest'. Worryingly, this same phenomenon is seen in patients who have a problem with their hearts, such as a heart attack or heart failure, and portends a poor outcome. What is particularly interesting is that the worse the depression, the worse the heart-rate variability.

Taking care of yourself

Thinking back to my patient in the clinic who was clearly depressed, one of the things that worried me the most was that he was still smoking. More importantly, he was still smoking because he told me he had absolutely nothing else to fill his days with.

On the wards, we have something we call the 'beard sign'. The first time I heard of this was when I was on my first term of cardiac surgery as a resident. We had a patient who was having heart surgery and going into it he was extremely sick. Unfortunately, after his surgery, he did not have a smooth recovery. He sat on our ward for close to six weeks, trying to get stronger every day, except that he couldn't because he was miserable from everything that had gone wrong. He just couldn't muster the effort to join in physiotherapy.

Funnily enough, one of the senior doctors predicted this. I remember him saying to me, 'Look, he's beard-sign positive, he's going to struggle.' What he meant was that this poor man had lost the will to do even the simplest things to take care of himself, like shaving his beard. I still remember the morning that we came into his room to find that he had shaved off the motley growth on his face – it was met with great fanfare. We intuitively knew this meant he was rallying, and as his body recovered, his mind did too. He went home not long after that.

Depression zaps all of your energy to do anything, especially take care of yourself. Living well or getting well requires a degree of commitment to a set of behaviours. Things like taking all of the medications you are prescribed, exercising, attending doctors' appointments and avoiding smoking or drinking. Aside from all of the biological factors at play, depression is also a direct impediment to being capable of getting out of bed and doing all of the things that are 'good for you'.

One study of patients who had heart disease looked not only at depression but also at motivation associated with depression. Exercise and cardiac rehabilitation is an important cornerstone to recovery after any kind of heart event. This particular study saw that in patients who were depressed, their motivation and subsequently their amount of exercise was very low compared to those who had no depression.

Anxiety often coexists with depression and is quite common in the general community. Using the same biological mechanisms and creating the same difficulties for patients to take care of themselves, anxiety adds to the risk of having a heart attack, and of having another heart attack after the first.

Healing hearts and minds

Depression is common. If we haven't had a period ourselves of feeling lower than low, then we probably know someone who has. And depression is now considered an important risk factor for a sick heart. The link between depression and heart disease is strong enough to have prompted professional heart powerhouses like the American Heart Association and the American College of Cardiology to write scientific statements on depression for respected heart-focused journals like *Circulation*.

We have medicines for blood pressure, and we can exercise and stop smoking. In more recent times, we also have medicines and treatments for depression. Depression needs to be treated not just for depression's sake but also because of the far-reaching consequences for the rest of the body. The wonderful thing about treating depression is that when the mind responds to treatment, the body becomes healthier too.

Antidepressants

Antidepressants such as Prozac and its many cousins are some of the most commonly prescribed medications around the world. With good reason. Prozac belongs to the class of drugs called SSRIs (selective serotonin reuptake inhibitors) that we discussed earlier. SSRIs provided a breakthrough in the treatment of depression and there's no doubt that they have saved lives. They are imperfect drugs but they have helped millions.

SSRIs have an important anti-inflammatory effect. They don't directly calm inflammation on the vessels and heart, but we believe they have some way of dropping the levels of pro-inflammatory cytokines and hormones in the bloodstream. In clinical trials, this hasn't always translated to a drop in rates of heart disease in depressed people. Most likely, the benefit of antidepressants on heart disease occurs when they are used at the same time as counselling and exercise programs. However, they probably help in getting people out of the slump that depression can induce so that they can fully engage in all of these other important treatments.

All antidepressants are not created equal. While SSRIs are highly prescribed and well known, there are many other classes of antidepressants. Getting the right antidepressant to treat depression is a difficult task as doctors and patients try to balance up benefits with side effects. In some people, the inflammation that puts them at risk of heart disease also impairs the ability of the antidepressants to work.

While antidepressants are and will continue to be very important tools in treating depression, they are no panacea. Exercise, however, *is* shaping up to be a one-stop shop for a number of illnesses. Exercise is an important treatment for depression and works by reducing inflammation and increasing the levels of neurotransmitters, or brain hormones, that lift our mood. The beauty of exercise is that it not only treats depression, it also has undeniably great effects on our heart health.

In a large study of patients with heart failure, an exercise program not only reduced the rates of patient hospitalisation for physical illnesses, but the rates of depression also dropped by as much as 10 per cent. In other studies, exercise as a treatment has a bit of an edge on antidepressants. Both are important features in treating depression, but exercise may be that little bit better.

There are many different formal counselling techniques or psychological therapies used to treat a variety of mental illnesses, including depression. The impact of counselling on treating depression and heart disease can be small, but is by no means insignificant or unimportant. Essentially, therapy and counselling are important parts of treating depression and providing life or psychological tools for the future.

While science may not yet show a distinct benefit in talking about our issues, we do know that suffering alone in silence is definitely not good for depression or our hearts. For a wide range of conditions, ages and social backgrounds, social isolation is a consistent predictor of not doing well health-wise. We can measure high levels of stress hormones like cortisol in people who are lonely or commonly experience high blood pressure. Both of these conditions can directly injure the heart. Social support is an important factor in being well, staying well and getting well when faced with illness. Remember my patient who came back to my clinic after his heart surgery? He had nobody to talk to; the doctors' appointments were his social outings.

Preventing the heart from being a casualty of the head

Plenty of work is being undertaken to look into the effects of depression on people who already have heart disease. This is despite the fact that we know that depression may set people up for developing heart disease down the track. Depression, anxiety and social isolation are now being considered alongside the more traditional risks for heart disease, such as diabetes. Being aware of these problems is one thing, but we need to think about prevention.

Firstly, being screened for, asking about and getting treatment for depression is extremely important; not just for your heart, but also for you as a person. For doctors and nurses, being attuned to the likelihood of someone having depression may allow us to act upon that elevated risk. The problem about risk is that unless we are shown black-and-white evidence that it is relevant to us or that it's already affecting us, we tend not to do much about it. Humans have an incredible knack for ignoring things for as long as possible.

Heart disease, by and large, does not happen overnight. It is a long, hard slog and depression contributes to that from earlier in our lives than we may realise. Recognising this early should prompt us to take better care of our hearts. Inevitably, better physical health will be rewarded with better mental health and will perpetuate good health.

Exercise seems to be a consistent factor in the prevention and treatment of depression, as well as heart disease. One major point we should all take away from this discussion is that exercise should be the number one thing we do for our health. Hand in hand with this is a healthy diet that maintains a healthy body weight, a healthy gut and a healthy brain by reducing the risk of obesity, inflammation, diabetes, depression and ultimately heart disease.

Finally, if negative emotions destroy our health, it should follow that positive emotions can improve it. Cultivate a life that makes you happy. Reach out for help and take care of your body. The power of developing true happiness helps your brain leave a positive mark on your physical health. Depression, anxiety and social isolation are not only making our day-to-day lives tough, they're also making us very sick. Take care of your whole self and the pieces will fall into place for a healthier, happier heart.

chapter 10
SLEEPY HEARTS

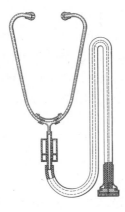

**I love sleep. My life has the tendency
to fall apart when I'm awake, you know?**
ERNEST HEMINGWAY, WRITER

I talk about sleep a lot more than the average person, I think. Most mornings on my ward rounds when I ask patients how they are, well over half say that they haven't slept. It's the hospital beds or the endless parade of machines that sing out at all hours. They often tell me they slept until they were woken up to have their observations checked by the nursing staff. Even though we all know the staff are just checking on them after major surgery, the frustration of interrupted sleep is easy to understand. Sometimes it's the nightmares and insomnia that can happen after major surgery, or the visits from little purple men, born of strong painkillers.

In fact, weird visions or nightmares from pain pills are not uncommon among my patients. I remember one elderly man telling me that after heart surgery he stayed up all night to chat to the green creatures sitting on his bed because, as he put it, 'they were bloody good company!'

Whatever the reason, there are few things more complained and worried about than a lack of sleep. It is disruptive and it makes you feel less than stellar – a kind of poor imitation of yourself. Sleep is said to solve everything from physical ailments to life's great questions. How many times have you been told that a good night's sleep will cure your cold or that maybe if you 'sleep on it', all of your problems will disappear? And the heart is front and centre when it comes to bearing the brunt of our modern lifestyle of too much work and too much play, or whatever it is that keeps you up at night.

Researching sleep has always been a little confronting for me, since in my job there are times when I have been incredibly sleep deprived, say when an emergency comes in. With a working week of 100 hours, being awake for days at time, and experiencing nights of sleep interrupted by phone calls and worry, I am acutely aware of the suffering sleeplessness induces in the body. (You'll be pleased to know that, although surgeons often work long hours, a number of scientific studies have demonstrated that we don't compromise our patients' outcomes. Especially not when someone needs us; we can still get the job done. Although after reading this research, I will try to make less of a habit of it!)

Hospital wards are filled with sleep-deprived patients. Illness may keep them awake or it may be the unfamiliar environment and huge numbers of medical machines that go ping. Sicker patients who are in intensive care develop a particularly dangerous type of sleep deprivation that can lead to delirium or even psychosis. The intensive care unit is a busy place 24 hours a day, and patients can have their internal body clocks become confused to the point that they don't sleep or they sleep at the wrong times.

Lack of sleep is something that is hard on a healing heart. These sleep-deprived patients are so tired that they feel every ache and pain more acutely than they would if they had had some rest. Their pain prevents them from getting better because they can't move and heal, and pain sets off all kinds of stress responses on the heart. Stress can show up on a monitor with a heart beating faster than it should – not a good way for a sick heart to be.

The adage that sleep fixes everything is not far from the truth. Sleep is restorative, it is vital and it is sadly lacking in modern life, and not just in the life of a surgeon. Increasingly we are appreciating that the quality and quantity of sleep that we have can play a vital role in our health and wellbeing, with the heart especially susceptible to sleep patterns.

A brief primer on sleep

What do you know about sleep? It is something we spend around a third of our lives doing, but is basically a magical, mystical occurrence that none of us know much about. Sleep seems like a short, static event: you go to sleep and then you wake up. Despite its simple appearance, sleep is incredibly nuanced.

There are two different types of sleep: REM and non-REM sleep. We need both types of sleep to feel refreshed and be healthy. REM stands for rapid eye movement. When we first go off to sleep, we enter non-REM or NREM sleep. NREM sleep progresses through several different stages until we reach REM sleep. We cycle through these two types of sleep all night and we can see when we're in each stage by taking an electrical recording of our brain activity.

The brain waves of electricity are faster in REM than in NREM sleep, but while the brain is busy, the body is doing absolutely nothing. We have no muscle tone but our eyes move rapidly in short bursts. The blood flow to our brains increases, as does our blood pressure. Dreams happen during this stage, which is why a kind of sleep paralysis is useful so we don't start acting out our dreams of flying or dancing or whatever our dreams are made of.

The brain is central to all of these parts of sleep, and the whole body changes when we sleep. We regulate body temperature differently during different parts of sleep, for example. Unsurprisingly, the heart and cardiovascular system change a lot when we sleep. For most of us, these changes are healthy and well tolerated; however, if you don't have all systems firing well, some of the heart and lung changes during sleep can place undue pressure on your heart.

Over the course of a good sleep, our heart rate slows, sometimes much lower than our resting heart rate. I am all too familiar with this one – it's not uncommon for me to receive a call from a worried doctor or nurse at 3 a.m. about a sleeping patient's heart rate that has fallen as low as 30. This slow heart rate occurs especially during NREM sleep, while in REM sleep it speeds up a little and varies a lot more, driven by our parasympathetic and sympathetic nervous systems.

During NREM sleep, the rest-and-digest parasympathetic nervous system is in charge. It fires off nerve signals that calm everything down – heart rate, blood pressure, even the force with which your heart beats. This is very good for your heart health as it means your heart is not working as hard as it usually does.

In addition to the nervous system, we have an in-built kind of clock called a circadian rhythm. Every living being has some kind of circadian rhythm, which the body generates through hormones and nervous system signals. It's the sleep–wake cycle that tells the body when to sleep and when to wake up. If you have ever travelled any great distance, it's the thing that jet lag destroys. Sunlight (or any light) and our daily activities modulate our internal body clocks. The circadian rhythm probably has a degree of influence over the way the heart behaves during sleep.

Waking up, especially naturally, is a process in itself. Waking happens when we get step-by-step activation in our sympathetic nervous system, which is the fight-or-flight arm. This causes our heart rate and blood pressure to rise just before we wake. The nervous systems also send messages to cause our adrenal glands to pump out cortisol, the stress hormone. Cortisol surging just before we wake up is thought to be our body gearing up for any stress we have to face in the day. Interestingly, more cortisol is produced when we wake up on a working day than on a weekend. This necessary surge in stress can be a bit of a strain on vulnerable hearts and it's one of the reasons that we see a spike in people having heart attacks first thing in the morning.

Naturally, over our lifetimes, our sleep patterns change. Newborns and infants begin with no regular rhythm, and sleep up to 18 hours a day. As they develop a circadian rhythm and are taught when to sleep with cues taken from feeding and environment, they sleep much more regularly.

Teenagers sleep more than adults, although few teenagers actually get the nine or 10 hours sleep that they need. Adults evolve their sleep patterns until older age when sleep quality tends to decline, which can place a lot of stress on the body.

Men and women sleep very differently. Men tend to be later to bed and later to wake. Women tend to wake up early and go to bed earlier. Women also struggle to get to sleep as easily as men and wake up more during the night, which can interrupt the restorative actions of a good sleep and place pressure on the heart.

Whatever your age, stage or individual need, sleep is an important part of your physical and mental health. Healthy sleep that keeps you feeling rested and alert during the day is associated with good health, especially for the heart. The heart needs sleep as much as the brain to repair and restore, as well as periods of rest and lowered blood pressure to give the heart and blood vessels a bit of reprieve.

Sleep has other benefits that can directly improve heart health. Healthy sleep helps regulate appetite, which in turn helps maintain a healthy body weight. It also helps our bodies respond to insulin more easily, which means they can store away sugar and fat that can directly hurt our hearts and blood vessels, staving off diabetes.

Bad sleep and bad hearts

Sickness can ruin your sleep. Any kind of illness, physical or mental, changes the equilibrium in your brain enough to make you sleep poorly or too little. In the case of my patients, heart surgery is such a big stress on the brain it can make them lie awake, eyes wide open, nearly all night. It's a phenomenon I always warn my patients about before their surgery.

When I was training in cardiothoracic surgery, I was lucky enough to learn from a wonderful mentor. That learning didn't stop at the operating theatre; he also taught me the valuable art of taking histories and getting consent from patients for surgery. Many years ago, I listened to him consent a patient for heart surgery, a coronary artery bypass graft procedure. I watched the patient describe the pain in his chest and go on to talk about his wife, who would take care of him after the surgery. My mentor then asked the man, 'You were a veteran, tell me about that.' The man's face dropped as he briefly mumbled something about Vietnam and how it 'wasn't that nice'. As we walked from the man's room, I asked my mentor why he was so interested in his service and he explained to me that when the brain is exposed to the stress of surgery, it can sometimes remember and dream about things it was trying to hide. Horrible things seen during war are an example of the memories your brain may try to forget, but the controlled trauma of surgery can cause you to remember.

Sure enough, after his surgery, the man slept badly. Not just badly – he was awoken repeatedly by flashbacks of war and suffering. The surgery and the stress to his body of the recovery afterwards produced bad sleep and terrible dreams.

The last time that you were feeling unwell, did you sleep well? Probably not. Sleep can be affected by upsetting the balance of a hormone called orexin. When orexin plummets in the brain due to illness, we sleep excessively, don't think as sharply and lose a little coordination in our arms and legs.

Inflammation is again at play when it comes to illness and poor sleep. A number of illnesses crank out inflammatory hormones, such as tumour necrosis factor (TNF). TNF can directly impact the brain and disrupt sleep. In patients who have just had heart surgery, TNF is high and so it may play a role in the poor sleep I warn my patients about.

Being sick can ruin your sleep, but what does ruined sleep do to your health? Are our health and especially our hearts at risk when it comes to sleeping badly? Given my tendency to be chronically lacking in sleep, this idea scares me. As it will probably scare many people, since a huge proportion of us are sleeping less, sleeping badly and are always exhausted.

The National Institutes of Health in the United States estimates that between 50 and 70 million Americans have a sleep disorder or are regularly sleeping poorly. Some people aren't sleeping well because of work (or play) commitments. Some have medical disorders that are responsible for poor sleep, such as obstructive sleep apnoea. Anxiety and depression also disrupt sleep patterns. All in all, we're tired and it's one of the worst things we can do to our hearts.

Snoring and snoozing

When it comes to sleep, the major culprits for sick hearts are insomnia or lack of sleep and obstructive sleep apnoea. Both are good at reducing the time asleep and the quality of sleep. Let's start with insomnia and plain old lack of sleep, since that's what a lot of us are suffering from. Insomnia comes in a few different forms. We can simply not sleep enough, for whatever reason. We can sleep in fits and starts, called fragmented sleep. Or finally, we can sleep what might be considered a reasonable number of hours but still feel tired and burnt out.

Insomnia is common, with some research papers finding that around 30 to 40 per cent of people report symptoms of insomnia over the course of a year. It can be the result of a medical condition or mental illness. Sometimes it's just regular life, whether that be work, a new baby or noisy neighbours. Insomnia seems to be more common in older people and in women.

A number of studies have looked at sleeping heart rates, comparing people with insomnia to people without. Consistently, these studies have shown elevated heart rates during sleep in those people with insomnia, which is thought to be driven by the stress hormones system, the hypothalamic-pituitary-adrenal axis. This axis is the set of cascading hormonal signals that exists between the brain, the pituitary gland at the base of the brain and the adrenal glands on top of the kidneys. This vital system starts when the brain tells the pituitary gland that we're stressed, which in turn tells the adrenal glands to pump out cortisol. We've met this stress hormone a few times now; it's useful when we're stressed acutely, but over the longer term, cortisol can go on a heart-unhealthy rampage.

Studying insomnia isn't straightforward and is often undertaken by questionnaire. The problem with these types of studies is that they can produce 'dirty' data, as it's difficult for any of us to recall accurately details about sleep. This has raised the question of whether the link found in some studies between poor sleep and high blood pressure is as strong as we thought. However, other large studies using more sophisticated methods and mathematical models have found having insomnia meant a person was 1.8 times as likely to have hypertension than someone who slept well. The hypothalamic-pituitary-adrenal axis and cortisol are wearing the blame here. Lack of sleep stresses our bodies and brains, so cortisol gets pumped out, thereby increasing blood pressure.

When researchers looked at people who either didn't get enough sleep a night or had difficulty falling asleep, the risk of developing any kind of heart disease was shown to almost triple in some studies. The reality is probably not as dramatic; however, with maths and extrapolation there is definitely some contribution from poor sleep (quality or time) to making our hearts sick.

What if we sleep normally most of the time but every now and again are seriously sleep deprived? Like when I went without sleep for a couple of days due to an emergency surgery. Acute sleep deprivation or sleep restriction feels awful. I have lost track of the number of times I've been so sleep deprived that I've understood why it is used as a method of torture. If you've ever been that tired, you'll know your body takes a huge hit: your muscles ache and you have a headache that will not go away. Our brains don't take sleep deprivation well. They get confused and uncoordinated, to the point where being awake for 16 hours and then getting behind the wheel of a car is the equivalent of driving with a blood-alcohol level of 0.08, above the legal limit in some places.

Studies have shown being sleep deprived isn't good for our hearts. Meta-analyses are a type of scientific study in which researchers pool together all of the data gleaned from many different and independent studies. The idea is to strengthen the positive parts of the study and minimise the weaknesses. Meta-analyses of heart disease and sleep deprivation show that sleep deprivation seems to correlate with heart disease. It also tends to lead to some of the risk behaviours, such as eating more and moving less, which then lead to an increased likelihood of developing diabetes, obesity or high blood pressure.

A study of Finnish women watched what happened when they were deprived of sleep for 40 hours. The women were hooked up to monitors to track how well they slept and how their hearts behaved. This study showed that particularly women who had gone through menopause had a reduced heart-rate variability, indicative of the autonomic system being overactive and causing the heart to work harder than it should. In these cases, over time the heart will start to show more 'wear and tear' from the extra work it's subjected to, which manifests as heart disease.

Aside from these specific changes in heart rate, the association of sleep problems with the precursors of heart disease is well established. Diabetes occurs around 30 per cent more in sleep-deprived people. Even a prediabetic state can occur as a result of sleep deprivation, whereby the body isn't as good at responding to insulin, leaving sugar to run around the bloodstream and damage tissues, including the heart and blood vessels. Blood pressure tends to climb, on average by around 13 mmHg, possibly leading to hypertension that, as we've discussed, is a big stressor on the heart and blood vessels.

A lot of us are running around exhausted nowadays. I find this data pretty scary because I am one of these tired people. There is another group of people who are not just tired but have a bona fide illness related to their sleep, and their risk is phenomenally high when it comes to hurting their hearts.

Sleep apnoea is a problem relating to the way a person breathes when they sleep. It's common too, with around 10 to 15 per cent of the population experiencing it. Apnoea is the medical term for when someone isn't breathing. In sleep apnoea, people stop breathing briefly multiple times throughout the night. When a sleep apnoea sufferer doesn't breathe, the levels of carbon dioxide rise in the body and are detected by receptors called chemoreceptors that tell the brain that it must not be breathing. The body is too clever to let that slide. Since the person is asleep though, the brain knows that the best and possibly only way to get them breathing again is to wake them up. Not fully, but enough to make them breathe again, and also enough to disrupt the quality of their sleep.

Sleep apnoea is diagnosed when someone has more than five of these little episodes of not breathing in an hour. This means that they are at least partially waking up around five times an hour. This is often associated with people who snore, because the same anatomy of the neck that causes snoring can also close off the upper airway and give rise to apnoea. We see it more in people who are overweight, because inevitably when any of us gain weight, some of it lands in the soft tissues of the neck. For others, it's just the way their airways are made that makes them prone to blocking off.

Sleep apnoea's effects on the heart start with the breathing issue. Not breathing is perceived as a big threat by the body, so all of our threat-related systems kick into gear to neutralise it. The sympathetic (fight-or-flight) nervous system drives blood pressure up, activates unhelpful hormone systems and tells our bodies that high blood pressure is okay. None of these processes are useful for the heart. The critical point is that a lack of breathing drives up blood pressure to levels that many studies say place far too great a strain on the heart. Over time, this leads to plaque forming in the arteries, the heart muscle getting dangerously stiff and large, and even rhythm problems with the heart, some of which can be fatal.

Treatment for sleep apnoea is generally centred on splinting the airway open with a machine called CPAP, which stands for continuous positive airway pressure. People with sleep apnoea wear a tight-fitting mask over their face or nose that looks kind of like an elephant trunk. It blows air into the nose, mouth and throat so that the pressure inside the airways is high enough to prevent them collapsing. CPAP machines were a turning point in treating sleep apnoea. On a walk around my ward you will usually find a few CPAP machines belonging to my patients. Using CPAP reduces the rates of heart disease and high blood pressure and, at a cellular level, it also affects how healthy the blood vessels are and even how much inflammation is happening.

The other cornerstone of treating sleep apnoea is weight loss. Reducing weight is a much cheaper and simpler way to tackle it, and has many added health benefits.

Does catch-up sleep help the heart?

Stepping inside my sometimes crazy world of work, I recall one weekend when I was operating or seeing patients for nearly 72 hours straight. I calculated that I had only had around three hours' sleep per night. So on my next day off, I slept a lot. While I felt physically better at the end of it, and that horrible headache went away, was it any good for my heart?

Research tells us you can't bank sleep. If I knew I was going to have a busy few days, I couldn't sleep more to charge myself for the upcoming sleep deprivation. When it comes to repaying sleep debt, it seems that regular sleep truly matters. Getting tired from work or play, then catching up on the weekends, is associated with an increased risk of heart disease. The best approach? Regularly sleeping well, catching up on sleep slowly and consistently, and taking care of your sleep all the time.

Sleeping to protect our hearts

Since catching up on sleep is not really beneficial, what does science tell us about getting a good night's rest? Research tends to agree that for most of us, the optimal amount of zzz's a night is around eight hours. Some people, such as teenagers and older people, need more than this. Some of us can function on and be healthy with less.

Although insomnia can occur independently of any other problem – physical, emotional or social – it's worthwhile seeing your doctor if sleep is a problem. Things to be on the lookout for include depression and anxiety, lung or heart problems (yes, they feed back on each other), diabetes or any condition that wakes you up all night. For example, arthritis that causes pain could wake you up regularly.

Achieving the number of hours you need is aided by a process called 'sleep hygiene'. Despite how that sounds, it's not about sleeping in a pristinely clean environment, but rather about getting a 'clean' sleep. There are things that we can all do to improve and maintain a good sleep, and they are particularly important if you have a tendency towards poor sleep.

Getting a regular amount of sleep enables us to feel rested, and waking up at a similar time every day helps our bodies to establish their body clock or circadian rhythm. If you, like me, lie awake staring at the ceiling as you try to force yourself off to sleep, get up and do something relaxing. Studies have shown that being awake worrying about sleep for longer than 20 minutes makes it even less likely that you will fall asleep. To reduce the likelihood of that happening, go to bed when you are actually sleepy.

Sleeping environment is also very important, and is affected by things like darkness, noise and temperature. Darkness causes the release of melatonin, which is your body's natural sleep hormone, so maintaining a dark room will help your body clock do its thing. This may come as no surprise, but our obsession with blue-light emitting screens like computers and smart phones is a big impediment to sleep. It actually confuses the natural body clock and makes the brain think it should be awake.

Exercise is also an important part of sleep hygiene, and should preferably be undertaken at least four hours before bedtime. That's not always possible, and any form of exercise, at whatever time you can do it, helps all the metabolic processes of your body behave normally. Even at a cell level, when everything works well, good sleep follows.

All these to-do's are well and good, but what about people like me who may need to be awake for long periods? What about shiftworkers or new parents? This may be the most challenging part of looking after our sleep, but this issue should be taken on as a public health measure. The US Army has taken this challenge in its stride, seeing sleep as a kind of 'secret weapon' to aid soldiers' performance and keep them mentally and physically healthy. It makes sure soldiers have the appropriate time and places to get proper sleep: it makes them much better at their jobs. Rosters that allow sufficient rest, or some much-needed quiet time for new parents being given by relatives or friends, is something we need to work into our culture, at work and at home. Sleep is far too important.

Modifying and enhancing work processes to allow for an appropriate rest time after the grind of the day is important for companies, but also for the health of us all. Can you get your business to have a no-after-hours email policy? Or perhaps introduce a strictly enforced finish time, unless there is a real emergency? Getting everyone on board may have an important role to play in making all of our hearts happier and healthier.

Employee wellness is not just something we should aim for in our workplaces because it's nice to look after each other. Don't get me wrong, it absolutely is and that should be reason enough. However, rested, happy and healthy employees tend to take less sick days and be more productive, which in turn means our organisations are more efficient and profitable.

chapter 11
FAMILY AFFAIRS OF THE HEART

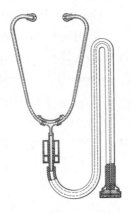

Your genetics is not your destiny
GEORGE M. CHURCH, GENETICIST
AND MOLECULAR ENGINEER

'I guess I have the genes for it,' was the explanation offered up by George. George was only 55 years old but had had a major heart attack that morning. His heart disease was so bad that he was in some ways lucky to be here talking to me about open-heart surgery. When I asked him what he meant, he proceeded to list off his three brothers who had all had coronary artery bypass grafting. One had three grafts, one had five, the other had three as well.

As we talked, one by one the brothers filed in, all exclaiming that they had been waiting for this for years now. They admonished George for not quitting smoking earlier. 'Sorry, but with your brothers all having had heart surgery, you still smoke?' I asked. George was a little sheepish and told me how many times he had tried to kick the habit, to no avail. I didn't need to tell him off, his brothers were already doing a great job of that.

George was partially right: with three out of his three siblings (plus their father) suffering heart attacks at early ages, his genetic make-up was not going to be favourable to having a healthy heart. They say you can't choose your parents, and perhaps this saying is actually directed at the genetic material you receive that you'd rather not have. I have inherited my mother's short-sightedness and my father's high blood pressure. They will both tell you I inherited their intelligence, to which I reply that I just studied hard!

We see a lot of family clustering of diseases, and it's well publicised that we need to understand what diseases 'run in the family'. It's a way of knowing what we might be up against. If a woman finds a breast lump and tells us her mother had breast cancer, we move that diagnosis further up the list. I know that high blood pressure and heart disease run in my family, so I checked these things sooner than I otherwise might have.

Having heart disease in your family is a red flag for doctors. When someone says their mum or dad had a heart attack, or heart failure, we automatically think that whatever is going on could be related to the heart. This is especially true if they were sick at a young age. Some of this influence comes from genes: what we've inherited. Some comes from the fact that, as a family, we often eat similarly or share similar activity levels – the environmental influence. Regardless of how bad your genes are, however, research shows a healthy lifestyle almost halves the likelihood of having a heart problem.

What are genes?

Let's take a step back and talk about what genes are. We often hear them mentioned in the media as a cause of some disease or a possible treatment. Most of us know that they're something that we get from our parents, and some of us know they have to do with DNA. But what is a gene and how does it cause disease?

DNA, or deoxyribonucleic acid, is the very basic building block of all of us. It's made up of four different compounds called **nucleotides** that always travel in pairs. The way these pairs organise themselves into a sequence forms a code that gives instructions to our cells on what to be, how to grow or what products to manufacture. A gene is a region of DNA that together will code for a particular process or structure in our bodies.

We all have two copies of every single gene, though they're not identical. Before we're born, we inherit half of our genes from each of our parents, which is why no set of two genes is necessarily the same. In some ways, this is nature's insurance policy of ensuring rare, recessive genes that may code for disease don't always replicate into the wider population.

These minor variations are a kind of mutation that occur through years of swapping genes with each other. It can also happen out of the blue, when a little bit of code changes spontaneously. A lot of the characteristics we share have arisen by a process of natural selection, whereby people with the most useful genes survived many years ago to pass on the so-called 'good genes'.

Genes code us. They are our blueprint from the time we're made, and throughout our lives. They can be turned on and off, depending on when they're needed or not needed. They build arms and legs when we're growing and tell our skin how much melanin to produce in the sun. They are at the heart of how everything works inside us.

Genes and disease

When it comes to disease, genes can be directly responsible. This might be the case when a gene is supposed to, say, build a kidney as per usual, but an error in the code means that it forgets to build two. The other way genes cause disease is by making us prone to hazards in our environment. So if our genes tell our bodies that high blood pressure is okay, our bodies won't take steps to reduce it.

Genetics can be complex and there is still a lot we don't know. The Human Genome Project set out to unravel the code of an entire human genome, that is a map of all the DNA codes in a body. After 15 years they sequenced 99 per cent of a human genome in 2003 and it formed the basis for future research into our genes.

The order of the code is one thing, but working out whether that order causes or even prevents disease is a bigger project. Researchers around the world use many techniques, including modifying the DNA of animals, to see what does what. A long and involved process involving years of research has enabled us to label specific genes, so that if a certain gene is seen, we know exactly what it does.

However, the story can get unbelievably complex. Just because someone has a gene for, say, heart disease doesn't necessarily mean that they will develop it. The first reason for this is that not every gene is turned on, or it might be overpowered by a stronger gene called a **dominant** gene. The overpowered gene is called **recessive**. This kind of single gene inheritance has been comprehensively researched, and tends to be associated with rarer diseases.

Another genetic reason is that for some diseases (heart disease included), there are multiple genes involved, some we haven't even discovered yet. In order for a person to get that disease, a critical number of genes need to be turned on. The genetic pathways that lead to heart disease also don't just affect the heart directly; they can affect how your body handles cholesterol or how prone you are to gaining weight.

The other important reason to keep in mind is that genes don't always equal disease. Our environment – such as nutrition, education or whether or not we smoke – can make genes more or less likely to be turned on. Or it can cause disease regardless of whether or not you are genetically predisposed to it. As we'll see, heart disease falls into this category.

The way I like to think of genes is this: you don't know for sure what genes you inherited from your parents, so assume the worst and take good care of yourself. You never know, you may be able to keep those 'bad genes' turned off.

The genetics of coronary disease

One of the difficulties of heart disease is that so many factors feed into it, causing blockages of the coronary arteries in the first place. Think of it as a multi-hit process: the arteries are bombarded by all kinds of environmental things like smoking, high blood pressure or high cholesterol. This all happens in the context of our genes, that tell our body how resistant, or not, they are to these insults. There are so many genetic predispositions for the risk factors of heart disease.

The complexity hasn't stopped people from looking for the genetic links in heart disease. Since 2007 around 50 different points in our genes have been identified as associated with heart disease. Some studies have identified up to 100. The risk is continuous – the more 'pro-coronary disease' genes a person has, the greater their risk of developing coronary artery disease.

The clue that genes could be at play came from years of epidemiological data. That is, looking at a large number of patients with heart disease and investigating who had it in their families, thereby allowing researchers to work out to what extent their genes betrayed them. They estimated that around 40 to 60 per cent of the susceptibility to heart disease was inherited. A big study called INTERHEART found that if someone in your family had heart disease, you were 1.5 times as likely to have heart disease yourself.

As we wrapped our heads around DNA, people went hunting for the genes that were responsible for heart disease. And there was a lot to be found. Researchers looked at huge numbers of people who had heart disease, took samples of DNA and worked out the code that made up each culprit gene. What they found was a vast array of genes that seemed to be associated with heart disease, because not all disease is governed by just one gene.

Many of us have some genes for various diseases. In fact, half the genetic variants that contribute to the risk of having a heart attack or angina are found in half the population. That means at least half of us carry a significant genetic burden to develop heart disease.

These individual genes themselves aren't disease-causing power-houses. On average, these genes increase your risk by around 18 per cent. Some genes only increase it by 2 per cent and some increase it as much as 90 per cent. A lot of the genes implicated in causing heart disease control other genes. They control when other genes are switched on or off. So, for example, one influential gene can instruct the cells to make too much of one product or too little. An inherited form of high cholesterol is a good example of this.

As we know, many problems feed into the development of heart disease. We see this quite strikingly in genetics, with 35 out of 50 known genes for heart disease acting on risk factors. These are genes that code for cholesterol management, blood pressure, diabetes or parts of the immune system that stir up the coronary arteries. Some genes act directly on blood vessel walls, making them slightly abnormal so they're more prone to developing atheroma or plaque.

When it comes to abnormal genes, not all are made equal. A gene called '9p21' seems to be particularly problematic. (The name 9p21 refers to the position in which we find the gene; some genes get fancier names than this.) This gene, when it's abnormal, weakens or damages the blood vessel so that plaque forms there. The more abnormal this gene is, the more severe the heart disease.

Another interesting genetic association is seen with blood groups. In the coding sequence determining our blood group (A, B, AB or O), lives a part of code that influences the stickiness of our blood. Blood stickiness or a tendency to clot is a problem in heart attacks because the blood sticks to plaque in the arteries, causing a sudden loss of blood supply to the heart muscle.

Some studies have shown that people with A or B type blood make a small protein that joins with another molecule called von Willebrand factor. Von Willebrand factor is important in blood clotting but once its job is done, it washes away. The protein that type A and B blood make keeps that factor hanging around for longer than it should, making the blood stickier and more likely to clot over any plaque that develops. This doesn't mean that you will have a heart attack based on your blood group; it may just add, even a little bit, to your risk of heart disease.

One study that could be placed in the basket of 'strange associations' found a link between short people and heart disease. Looking at 200,000 people of European descent, the study showed that people who had genes for being shorter also had more coronary artery disease. Seems odd, but researchers found that the genes that code for height were also working on blood cholesterol and triglycerides. While those genes were making people shorter, they were also shooting their cholesterol up.

Another important area of genetic study that will no doubt develop further relates to statins, which are a group of drugs used to lower cholesterol. People with a higher burden of genes considered bad for them have been found to gain more benefit from statin therapy. Their cholesterol dropped, as did their rates of heart disease by nearly half. The discovery of genes may mean we can target who we treat and with what drugs.

An important and very common disease that greatly increases the risk of heart disease is familial hypercholesterolemia. People with this disease have extremely high levels of LDL (bad) cholesterol and as a result, they develop blockages to their arteries much younger than other people. Some have heart disease and heart attacks before the age of 20. They inherit one of three genes that prevent LDL from binding to its receptor to be taken out of the blood, instead causing it to float around and damage the blood vessels.

Are there any protective genes? Absolutely. In fact, the way your body responds to exercise may be influenced by your genes: genetic variants allow some people's body fat to drop more easily with exercise than others. This may be involved in decreasing the risk of heart disease.

Using genetic risk predictions, we may be able to predict how likely someone is to develop heart disease and possibly work out who is at risk early on, before they develop the disease. Equations that look at age, gender, blood pressure and cholesterol, as well as family history, can give an estimate of how likely someone is to have a heart problem in, say, 10 years.

Despite the benefits, genetic testing has a bit of a dark side. It remains quite expensive. In countries where this cost is borne by patients and their families, the potential benefits may not be accessible. And access to genetically targeted treatments might be precluded without the appropriate testing.

Another drawback relates to insurance. If insurance companies could access our genetic blueprints and see what diseases we were likely to get, they may limit our cover for those diseases. The same goes for life insurance. It's a potentially discriminatory and ethically loaded conversation.

All in all, the genes for heart disease are complicated and there's continual work being done to obtain more information. Whether that leads to targeted drugs or earlier screening remains to be seen. The most important point to remember is that genes at best account for around half of your risk. The rest is up to each and every one of us.

Genetically linked heart diseases

The first cardiac disease to have its genes identified was familial hypertrophic cardiomyopathy. This was soon followed by other disorders related to heart rhythm disturbances that leave people prone to sudden cardiac arrest. A number of these diseases have a specific gene associated with them rather than the dozens or more that influence coronary artery disease.

I met a patient once who knew all too well that genes can make the heart extremely sick. He was in his early forties and lived a very clean life. He had no choice. In his family, multiple people had a severe form of heart disease called dilated cardiomyopathy. We sat talking in his room about placing a mechanical heart; he was waiting for a heart transplant but had become too sick. His brother sat with him. He had the telltale scar down the centre of his chest from open-heart surgery. He had undergone a heart transplant for the same condition four years earlier. Their father had died very suddenly in his late thirties. It was a family legacy – one none of them wanted.

Dilated cardiomyopathy is a disease of the heart muscle that causes it to stretch and the heart to become big and baggy. It doesn't pump well and people with this disease develop severe heart failure. Around a third of the genes that are found with this type of heart disease make abnormal cells that fail. Genetics aren't the only cause of this heart muscle disease, but when we screen the relatives of people who have it, a number of them share genes that cause it.

One reason the genetics of dilated cardiomyopathy are so important is that we can detect if anyone else in a family is at risk. If they are, we can keep a close eye on them and provide early treatment. Another reason is that the genes for this disease are 'strong'. Most of the genes that code for it are dominant, so you only need one copy from either parent to develop it.

Hypertrophic cardiomyopathy is another common type of heart muscle disease, but rather than getting stretched and baggy, these hearts pump up like a body builder's biceps. The heart gets so big it can't effectively pump blood out because it's obstructed. The coronary arteries struggle to keep up with the enormous muscle mass, so they can have lots of small and silent heart attacks.

One of the more worrying features of hypertrophic cardiomyopathy is that it can lead to dangerous heart rhythms, causing the heart to stop abruptly. It's the most common cause of sudden death in young athletes. A number of sports programs around the world screen all of their athletes for it.

Between 60 and 70 per cent of people with this disease carry genes that cause abnormal heart muscle cells. There are around 15 different genes that code for this disease and again, screening is important among the family of anyone who has it.

During my time working in paediatric cardiac surgery, I saw a number of patients with a disease called long QT syndrome. One child specifically sticks in my mind. She was only 10 years old and had been playing in the schoolyard at lunchtime when she slumped to the ground. Thankfully, quick-thinking teachers began resuscitaton. When an ambulance arrived, paramedics placed monitors on her little body and saw that she had a very dangerous heart rhythm called ventricular fibrillation, whereby the heart doesn't pump, it shakes. Using electrical pads on her chest they tried to shock her heart back to normal, but it didn't work. She arrived at our hospital where we placed her on a heart–lung machine while other doctors worked at getting her heart into a normal rhythm.

The heart muscle contracts to its own electrical system by ions moving in and out of the cell. As they move, they transfer charge, or electricity, and make the cell contract. Kind of like if you were unfortunate enough to touch an electric fence, your arm muscles would contract. In people with long QT syndrome, the tiny channels these ions flow in and out of are not quite normal so the electrical activity of the heart is prone to serious upset.

Being able to screen other family members for this disease means that we can treat them before they collapse. Our genetic testing later revealed this little girl's younger brother had the genes, and they both received internal defibrillators so that if their heart rhythms became dangerous, they would immediately get a shock to save their lives.

The tough aspect of these inherited types of heart disease is that they're difficult to sidestep if you have the genes. However, the study of genetics has brought us the ability to hone in and make drugs that specifically target the product of a gene. For example, a drug has been developed to target one of the defective proteins in familial hypercholesterolemia. While no such drugs exist yet for these other conditions, it's something that we could possibly achieve in the future and is considered the holy grail of working out genes and their pathways.

Nurture

Genetics isn't the only thing that we can thank our parents for. In a process called programming, it is mothers who are the influencing factor. The theory behind programming is that if we're exposed to something in the uterus, it sets up processes in the body that affect us for the rest of our lives. Over the last few decades, a lot of research has been directed at what happens to us before we're born and how that sets us up for heart disease or other problems in adult life.

Most of this research came out of a finding many years ago that babies who were born very underweight went on to develop heart disease at higher rates than babies who weighed more. The question was then asked: what is it that happens before birth that impacts on disease throughout life?

High levels of cholesterol in a mother's pregnancy can affect a person in childhood and adulthood. If a mother has high cholesterol, her children have early plaque formation at rates above kids whose mothers have normal cholesterol. Cholesterol can't cross the placenta – it's too big a molecule. But it is believed that the chain reaction that cholesterol causes in a mother, including inflammation, is what sets the process off in her baby.

The babies of smoking mothers are at risk of many problems, including poor growth. Smoking is associated with high blood pressure inside the umbilical vessels and foetal brain blood vessels, and poor flow in the foetal aorta. Given all the nutrition a growing baby needs, this high blood pressure impedes the vital delivery of nutrient-rich blood to the baby. We see that these babies grow up to have thicker than normal carotid arteries in their necks, which is strongly associated with developing heart disease.

When a mother is carrying too much extra weight or has diabetes, a baby can be affected in the womb. These babies often have a larger than normal birth weight. Very large babies may have abnormal blood lipids, or fats, that cause damage to the blood vessels over life. These babies and their mothers are also at higher risk of complications during the pregnancy; some can be extremely dangerous for them both. The babies can also have high blood pressure at birth, which can stick around for long enough to cause heart problems.

A bit like genetics, just because a mother smoked or had high cholesterol does not necessarily mean that a disease will occur. It's also unfair to attribute whatever happened in pregnancy to what happens throughout the rest of somebody's life. The steps that go into creating disease of the coronary arteries that causes heart attacks happen over many years in a gradual process. There are straightforward influences that we can change, like smoking for example, but the rest of it is far more complex. For now, ensuring expectant mothers stay as healthy as possible is good for them, good for their babies and probably good for the rest of their lives, too.

Can you fight your genes?

We love to shrug our shoulders and say it's in our genes. Whether it be our bad taste in music or something more serious such as heart disease, the general feeling is that once Mother Nature has gifted you the blueprints for disease, fighting back is hard. Like George, the patient we met earlier, who had come to the decision that you can't fight your genes: it can't change things anyway. Or can it?

In 1948 an ambitious study of heart health, called the Framingham Heart Study, was launched. It enrolled 5209 residents of Framingham, Massachusetts, and followed them for their life-times. The researchers watched what happened to them over time and tried to match what happened or what they did to the presence or absence of heart disease. Huge amounts of important information were discovered with this study, some of which contributed vital clues in the fight against heart disease.

The researchers didn't stop there though. In order to study how family factors and genetics influenced heart disease, the Framingham Study went on to recruit the next two generations – the vast majority related to the first cohort. Not only did they watch what happened to these people, they had gathered the DNA of thousands of participants.

In the Framingham Study, genetic determinism or yielding to our genes isn't supported. That is to say, our genes are not responsible for *all* of our destiny. They are definitely a part of the story of who we are and who we become, but when it comes to heart disease, these epidemiological studies have demonstrated quite clearly that there is a complex interplay between our genes and the environment. What we do to or for our bodies matters.

Another important study, published in 2016, served as an important wake-up call against resigning yourself to genetic fate. This study took the DNA and all the clinical and lifestyle data of multiple cohort studies like Framingham. It tested the participants for the 50 known genes associated with heart disease. These results were then put into an equation that predicted heart disease to give an estimate of likelihood based on a person's genes.

The researchers then looked at two other factors. The first was: did they get heart disease? Did they have a heart attack, did they need heart surgery or stenting or did they die of heart disease? Then they matched all of this to the most important lifestyle factors: smoking, obesity, physical activity and diet, mainly looking at how much fish and vegetables a person ate.

The results were striking. This was a key study that showed even if you had lots of genes for heart disease, making healthy choices nearly halved the chance of heart disease. Even in the group dealt the worst hand of genes and the highest risk, this halving of heart problems was seen. In this high-risk group, after 10 years 10 per cent of people who didn't take good care of themselves had heart attacks. Compare this with just five per cent of high-risk people who did look after their hearts. The other notable finding was that the more healthy things you did, the more your risk was reduced.

When it comes to nasty disorders like familial hypercholesterolemia, the evidence isn't as strong. However, in this group of patients who already have an incredibly high risk of heart issues, adding insult to injury with smoking, diabetes or obesity markedly increases their risk. While the data looking at what happens if they avoid all of these things isn't conclusive, the feeling is that managing their lifestyles is an important tool for health.

Being a slave to your genes isn't necessarily something you have to do. In conditions such as coronary artery disease, the interaction between our genes and our environment is complex, which is a gift. It's a gift to be able to turn your genetic destiny on its head. If, like at least half of us, you have those genes or family history that puts your heart at risk, your challenge is to take extra special care of it, because science tells us that it is worth the effort.

chapter 12
HOW TO TALK ABOUT YOUR HEART

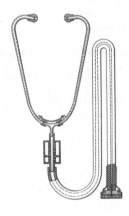

He who studies medicine without books sails an uncharted sea, but he who studies medicine without patients does not go to sea at all
WILLIAM OSLER, PHYSICIAN

In medicine, the art of history taking is like encouraging someone to tell their own story. Most of the time it's just listening, and in that listening, the answers appear. Sometimes it's gently guiding a patient to share the intricacies of their own story so that together we can work out what comes next. From very early on in medical school we're taught how to listen and coax. The gift for being good at this part of being a doctor is that if you listen closely, the patient leads you to their diagnosis. It's a skill that we hone for years.

As a junior doctor, I was rotating through a term in the emergency department. This is where storytelling is most important because the first time you meet someone, there are no tests to do the work for you; you need to ask and listen and be guided. An elderly gentleman had been brought in by ambulance. At the end of his bed the chart read, 'Brought in by ambulance. Daughter says more confused' in the standard, directed half-sentences healthcare workers use to save space and time.

I walked into his cubicle, introduced myself and then committed the error of asking, 'What brought you into hospital today?' He looked at me like I was a complete idiot: 'Well, the ambulance!' Not learning from my mistake, I asked, 'Why did you call the ambulance?' and he, again frustrated by my daft questions, said, 'I didn't call the ambulance! My daughter did!' I took the bait once more: 'Why did your daughter call the ambulance?' He again became frustrated and replied: 'I don't know! You'll have to ask her!'

The great physician Sir William Osler, who insisted on the importance of talking and listening to patients, believed that doctor and patient needed to communicate well with one another, or they risked falling short of what was needed and wanted. Navigating the healthcare system can be daunting at the best of times. It is complex, diseases can be complex, treatments are complicated and we are all rushed for time. The healthcare system also exists outside of hospitals and doctors' offices, and talking about health in our communities is very important. Developing the language and confidence to talk about our bodies or healthy behaviours may enable us to strip away some of the secrets around healthcare.

Talking about health

Women's heart disease is a big secret. Almost 10 years ago the Australian Heart Foundation set out to raise awareness and began by asking a simple question to women: did they think that heart disease was personally relevant to them? That is, did they need to worry about it? At the beginning of this campaign to raise awareness of the leading killer of women, a paltry two out of 10 women thought that they needed to be bothered about heart disease. Even after nearly 10 years of work, women still aren't receiving the message that hearts are important. Nowadays, only three out of 10 Australian women think that heart disease is a problem they need to worry about.

Aside from our day-to-day interactions with people around us at work or in our personal lives, social media and social networking websites link us to more people than ever before. Far from simply being a platform to share cat videos or family photos, social media shows tremendous potential when it comes to health. One of the possible strengths of online forums is to be able to promote health, whether through disseminating health information or by providing support from peers or online 'coaches'. Weight loss is a great example of an online peer group that can be used to provide both information and support. Some online communities even link scientists and doctors with patients. Breast cancer in social media (#bcsm) and lung cancer in social media (#lcsm) are two great online entities where patients and doctors join together for a common goal.

Generally, when we look at online or social media–based health interventions, linking in with like-minded people online is very useful for providing education, social support and tools to manage our own health. Research is now assessing how useful it is to get that peer-group support, but the belief is that this kind of interaction has great potential for creating healthy behaviours.

The incredible benefits of talking about health were evident in a recent US study published in the *Annals of Internal Medicine*, specifically looking at diabetes. This caught my eye, since diabetes is such a core issue in patients with heart disease. The study focused on a highly vulnerable group when it comes to diabetes – African Americans. Their diabetes tends to be less well controlled and they experience more diabetes-related complications, including heart disease and kidney disease.

This study pitted a financial incentive to get these patients taking care of their diabetes against peer support. They matched people who were struggling to take care of their diabetes with others who were managing their diabetes more successfully. The group receiving mentorship from a fellow diabetic got their blood sugars under much better control than the people who were paid to do it. This was a great example of the effects of getting a conversation started and how establishing a sense of camaraderie can strengthen health resolve.

Another example of the importance of this kind of peer support was discussed in a wonderful column I read in *The New York Times* by surgeon Dr Pauline Chen, who writes about doctors and patients. She told the story of a gentleman awaiting a liver transplant. Understandably, he was incredibly worried: whether he would get a liver in time, how he would cope with the surgery and whether or not he had the physical and psychological reserve to make it. Chen wrote: 'In desperation, he told me, he had contacted several patients who had already undergone a transplant. "That's what made me believe I'd be OK," he said. "You doctors have answered all of my questions, but what I really needed was to hear the stories about transplant from people like me."'

At my hospital, our patients on LVADs who are awaiting surgery are put through their paces at our cardiac rehabilitation gym. They're there to get strong and stay healthy while they wait for a transplant, working out harder than a lot of us do. A side effect of their exercise is that they do it together, swapping stories and sharing support. Being in that gym and watching them help each other, it became evident to me that their shared knowledge and fellowship in this very unique club was every bit as important as what we healthcare workers had to say.

Whether it's sharing our stories with each other in social media support groups, in a rehabilitation gym or via mass education campaigns like those the Heart Foundation uses, knowledge is power. Taking our discussions of heart health out from behind closed doctors' doors or from whispered conversations about someone's 'broken ticker' empower us all to get curious and get serious about taking care of our precious hearts.

Bill's story

I was just about to start operating one Thursday morning. One of our cardiologists opened the door of the operating theatre and said, 'Need you in cath lab, right now!' She didn't have to say more – that usually meant a cardiac arrest and that we needed to put the patient on a heart–lung machine in order to save them. Our whole room knew it was an emergency.

I ran down a few corridors to the cardiac catheter lab. I found Bill, only 60 years old, whose heart had stopped in the emergency department. He had woken up that morning with chest pain but had gone to work where it worsened, and so, scared of what it meant, he called an ambulance. His heart had stopped for more than 30 minutes; he was being kept alive by a machine pushing on his heart and a breathing tube working for his lungs. He wasn't getting better though, so we needed something more serious.

My team and I worked quickly and put two large pipes into the blood vessels in his groins. The blood filled the tubing of the heart–lung machine and took over the work of his damaged heart. He was stabilising but was still extremely sick. An ultrasound of his heart was concerning: it was hardly moving and had a dangerous rhythm. A team of over a dozen doctors and nurses raced to find and fix the problem.

Cardiologists injected dye into his coronary arteries and the cause jumped out at us on the screens above out heads. He had suffered an enormous heart attack, severely damaging the heart. The cardiologists opened up the blocked vessels with tiny stents. As blood flowed back down the coronary arteries, his heart began to beat in a more orderly way.

Back in the intensive care unit, his devastated family listened as various doctors explained what had happened and what would happen next. His daughter said through sobs, 'I told him, I told him to stop smoking and to see his doctor weeks ago!' She said that he had experienced a 'niggle' in his chest, which she had wanted him to get checked out. He didn't; instead he got to meet all of our team in a hurry. (Happily, he made a slow, but steady recovery. And gave up smoking successfully.)

On the lookout: symptoms and how to talk about them

A niggle or a pain; what is it that you should be looking for? Are there symptoms that you shouldn't ignore? It seems so often that heart disease creeps up on us, but there are definitely things you should be keeping an eye out for. These are the symptoms that can give you clues that there might be a problem with your heart and that it needs to be checked.

* *Chest pain: This is the classic symptom we are told to keep an eye out for. One man described this pain to me as 'like an elephant sitting on your chest'. Pain usually in the centre of the chest is a sign of the heart muscle not having enough oxygen, not unlike your muscles in your legs when you exercise. Generally, it happens when the heart has to work harder – walking up a flight of stairs for instance. Sometimes the pain can travel or radiate to other*

places, like to the back, neck or arms. In women especially, that
pain can be unusual or atypical and can start in the jaw or back.
* Short on puff: Some people with heart troubles feel a little like
they're running a marathon all the time. If your heart is sick,
whether in the coronary arteries or a valve, it cannot keep up
with what your moving body needs. Shortness of breath can
come on slowly, but if you can't keep up what you used to do,
it's definitely time for a visit to your doctor.

If you feel short of breath, especially when lying flat, that's
another kind of breathlessness we want to know about. Sick
hearts let fluid back up into the lungs and when you lie flat,
it makes you cough and gasp for breath.
* Swelling: When the heart can't pump well, there is back pressure
that builds up all the way down to your ankles, making them
swell up markedly. Think of how swollen your feet can get at the
end of a day, especially if you've been standing. That multiplied
several times is the kind of swelling we're talking about.
* Palpitations: Being abnormally aware of your heartbeat,
especially if it feels fast or irregular and this sensation doesn't
go away, signifies the need for an appointment with the doctor.
If you feel really awful while it's happening, or short of breath,
then you need a visit to the hospital. When this happens, you
can take your pulse at your wrist – just under your thumb is the
radial pulse. Is it regular and fast? Or is it irregular? If you're
able to get to the doctor while it's happening, we may be able
to catch it on a heart monitor and make a diagnosis.
* You're worried: Being worried is a good enough reason to get
checked out. Sometimes we just know when something isn't
quite right in our bodies. Whether it is a little pain or you feel
exhausted all the time, have a chat to your doctor. Even if what
you're feeling is just a little worried or anxious, that in itself is
OK to talk to your doctor about.

What is a heart health check?

A heart health check is a basic once-over by a doctor or experienced nurse to work out your personal risks for heart disease. It should always start with a chat about your heart, looking for symptoms, talking about your family and what things you do for (or sometimes against) your heart. It's a great opportunity to talk about smoking or weight loss, if they are issues that you're concerned about.

The physical part of the check is geared to looking at your weight. We've touched on how BMI (body mass index) can be a blunt tool, but a waist-to-hip ratio may be useful. Your blood pressure should be checked and doctors can do a spot check of your blood sugar. Finally, a blood test to check the lipids or fats in your blood is important. Generally, this is done when you've fasted so that it isn't falsely high from whatever you have had to eat (even if it was 'low fat').

Who should be getting a heart health check? Most research and heart health groups say anyone over 45 years old. For the most part, that's probably reasonable. However, everyone should know their blood pressure. Most women who take the oral contraceptive pill have their blood pressure checked annually when they have their prescription refilled.

During random screening for Stroke Week in Australia, a whopping 38 per cent of men and 26 per cent of women had high blood pressure. It's a test that takes literally a minute and since high blood pressure is completely without symptoms most of the time, the only way to know is to roll up your sleeve and have it checked.

The other important group to be checked is new mothers, especially those who had high blood pressure or diabetes during pregnancy. We know that women who have had these issues have a much greater risk of developing diabetes, high blood pressure or heart disease down the track. If you are one of these people, I recommend making it a habit to be checked each time your baby is checked.

Finally, these are also screening tests for people who don't have symptoms. If you know you're at high risk of heart disease, or have some symptoms, then you have every reason in the world to see your doctor even before you hit 45 years of age.

We don't yet have a magical test that can work out how likely it is that a person who is otherwise fit and well will have heart troubles. Tests like electrocardiograms (ECG), echocardiograms (ultrasounds) or computerised tomography (CT) coronary angiograms have minimal utility in people who appear healthy according to our standard risk assessments. The biggest problem with these tests is that they may not be able to show very early heart disease. In the case of CT, the problems of radiation exposure or allergy to X-ray dye can be added to that false reassurance.

The whole idea is prevention

Just like my patient Bill, whose daughter had urged him to visit the doctor a week earlier, we all want to prevent or at least minimise heart disease well before it takes hold. The whole idea behind knowing about your heart is to work towards making it as healthy as it can possibly be in the first place. Or if you have a heart problem, to try to fix that before you have a more serious problem like a heart attack.

Prevention comes from knowledge. So, armed with your new heart knowledge, start the conversation. Tell people about how incredible their hearts are and how they can look after them. Tell your doctor that you really care about your heart health and that you want to make it as strong as it can possibly be. Tell yourself that you are worth the effort.

Talking to your doctor: getting your message across

None of us should ever underestimate our intimate knowledge of ourselves. Years ago, this wasn't often appreciated. The doctor–patient relationship was doctor-led and doctor-dictated; the patient was expected to come along for the ride. Patients often deferred wholly to their doctor, and in many ways this led to a rather paternalistic relationship. I remember being taught anatomy by a very old surgeon who told me that when he first started working as a doctor, his word was gospel and that was all.

Thankfully times have changed. We are not here just to fight disease, and there is no 'them' (patients) or 'us' (doctors). We have now moved to what we call patient-centred care. It's not about ignoring the judgement of doctors, nor is it ignoring the patient, but rather we're all in it together. We're not fighting a disease; we're helping a patient who happens to have a disease.

Visiting a doctor or a hospital can be a daunting thing to do. We've all been there: you're embarrassed, you feel silly, you don't want to waste anyone's time. You may be afraid you won't be taken seriously – perhaps that is what has happened in the past. There's jargon and tests and confusion added to the fact that you are worried about whatever it is that has taken you there in the first place.

When it comes to your health, your experience is irreplaceable. Your symptoms, your worries – no tests will surpass those things that are very personal to you. Share them as openly as you can, including how much they worry you. It may be a piece of the puzzle that helps make a diagnosis or it may be something that you can be reassured about, relieving your anxiety. The more openly you share your own experience, the better the information that we can use to work out what is going on.

It goes both ways, too. As doctors, we should listen to you and share information freely. It's my job to explain to you what is wrong with your heart so that you can understand, to let you ask questions and answer them as best I can. If I don't know the answer, it's my job to find out for you. It's also my job to understand that you don't have time to be sick, and to help you plan how your life outside the hospital walls is going to continue.

What if you feel like you're not being heard? It's a real problem for a number of people. I've even sat across from a doctor myself and wondered if she heard a word that I said. It's not a great feeling. I look back at that experience and I felt really small, frustrated and worried that we may have missed something important.

What can you do to help get your message across? Speak up for your body and your health. Say what you're worried about and why and then listen to the explanation that you're given. Sometimes it helps to have someone else with you, especially when it's about something serious, like your heart. When you're worried, you remember half – probably at most – of what you're told. It is very useful to write notes; I'm a big fan of writing down things I need to remember and when my patients do, I know we're both getting our messages across.

Navigating the healthcare system can be daunting for anyone. Find a doctor you trust and respect and be your own heart advocate. The best way we can keep your heart healthy is if we do it together. Speak up and ask for what your heart needs. It's far too precious not to.

chapter 13
THE HEART'S JOURNEY: WHERE WE'VE COME FROM AND WHERE WE ARE GOING

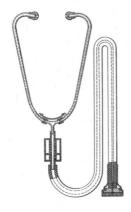

The time to repair the roof is when the sun is shining

JOHN F. KENNEDY, AMERICAN PRESIDENT

The story of the heart and those who work on it is quite something. Despite the technology now available, the bravery of patients and the ingenuity of researchers, it's important to keep in mind that prevention is still the best medicine. But as rates of heart disease continue to rise around the world, the best and brightest minds are working on ways to save broken hearts.

It's hard to believe that heart surgery has only been around for 60 years or so. The same could be said for most of modern medicine. Almost every day we hear about something phenomenal that provides new tools to fight disease. From relatively recent beginnings, the science and medicine of the heart have evolved rapidly, and continue to do so.

Where it all began

Heart surgery did not exist until the middle of the twentieth century. Before then, the only real option was to sew heart wounds as quickly as possible before a patient perished. Countless people who were born with or developed heart disease died from it, as doctors had no technology, no means to fix it.

It wasn't through a lack of trying though. One example of early medical ingenuity was a hole-plugging technique surgeons used to treat holes in the hearts of children who had turned blue from a lack of oxygen. The early surgeons would open up their patient, locate the hole with their finger and sew around it as quickly as possible. Many patients, unsurprisingly, did not make it through this surgery.

It wasn't until the late 1950s and 1960s that a group of heart surgeons from Minnesota began to work on ways to essentially still the heart so that they could repair it. They first began with a technique called cross-circulation in which, in the ultimate act of love and altruism, a parent would act as a kind of heart–lung machine for their child. Connected to one another by tubes, the parent kept the child alive. To this day, heart surgery facilitated by cross-circulation remains one of the few operations with a potential 200 per cent mortality.

At the same time that cross-circulation was at centre stage, groups of surgeons in Minnesota, Philadelphia and Boston were hard at work building the first heart–lung machines. The cardio-pulmonary bypass machines were enormous and took blood from a patient, added oxygen and returned it to the patient. At the same time, surgeons had been practising the art of stopping the heart from beating and then restarting it. This meant that heart surgery could finally be performed on a still, bloodless heart and patients could have a chance of being cured. Later that decade, the first heart transplant was performed on a man called Louis Washkansky by a surgeon called Christiaan Barnard in Groote Schuur hospital in Cape Town, South Africa.

From the late 1960s, heart surgery exploded. Medical conditions that were once universally fatal became conditions that could be treated. Lives were saved; lives were improved. The fact that all of this happened only 50 years ago is extraordinary. When I have talked to my senior colleagues over the years, they have told me that when they were teenagers, the occupation of heart surgeon did not even exist. In the last 50 years or so, the way we treat the heart has progressed and evolved in many ways and continues to do so.

When I first started in cardiac surgery as a very junior doctor, I was in awe of everything, but transplants were particularly interesting to me. I found it endlessly fascinating that it was possible to remove someone's heart and replace it.

In my first weeks on the service, there were two transplant patients who were supported on VADs, the mechanical hearts we explored earlier. One was connected via pipes from the heart, through his belly to a console that drove the pump. It made a huge whooshing noise as compressed air operated the pump. After his transplant, he missed the constant noise of the console because, he explained, 'When I heard it, I knew that I was alive'.

Ten years in this specialty is a relatively short time but changes in the way we take care of hearts have occurred continuously. We learn more and more every day and are able to tackle challenges that were previously out of reach. The heart is not particularly skilled at healing itself at the moment: damage tends to be permanent. Dreams of having a heart heal itself completely were once far-off, but these hopes are now becoming reality. They have moved from if, to when.

If we were to look into the future, what might we see when it comes to our hearts? Will heart transplants be a thing of the past? Will heart disease be eradicated by a pill or a vaccine? Will public health changes such as a sugar tax have the same effects as tobacco control? Or as our waistlines continue to grow, are we headed for a catastrophic spike in heart disease?

Stem cells and zebra fish

As far back as 2001, the British Heart Foundation was using zebra fish to heal hearts. It sounds a bit of a stretch. On the surface, we are very different to these beautiful tropical fish. But in reality, not only do we have more in common than meets the eye, we desperately want something that zebra fish have: their ability to regrow a damaged heart.

The human heart is so precious that if you irreversibly injure the cells of the heart, they die. And when they die, that's it: they can't regrow; they can't regenerate. I've seen many hearts that have been irreversibly damaged, usually from a heart attack. The area of the heart that has been badly damaged is a tough white patch of scar tissue. Just as a scar forms when you cut your skin deep enough, the same happens on the heart.

The biggest disadvantage of scarring is that it contributes nothing to the pumping action of the heart. And once it's there, it's there to stay. It won't change back to healthy heart muscle with time or tablets. Once the damage is done, it is done. Humans evolved to be clever with hands that are dexterous, and big brains. We socialise and farm and walk on two feet. One thing we forgot to evolve was the ability to heal our hearts when they were badly damaged.

Zebra fish and humans share quite a large amount of DNA; in fact, we have some very similar genes. An enormous amount of research is being undertaken to work out how we can switch on the genes in humans that zebra fish use to regenerate and repair their damaged hearts. At the moment, the repair genes in our hearts aren't switched on properly. When the heart is damaged, the repair mechanisms are more like a bandaid over a gash: it partially relieves the problem but it isn't exactly as good as new.

The rest of our bodies aren't like that. The lining of our gut can regenerate and our blood cells are turned over a little more often than once a month. These tissues do this by a process of maturation from precursor cells. These cells are like infantile versions of the various cells of the body. There are precursor blood cells, for example, that start to mature into their final form when they are exposed to various hormones.

Stem cells are often in the news as a potential cure for many illnesses and injuries. A stem cell is a unique type of cell that is not yet specialised as a skin cell or a heart cell, for example. They are able to form into nearly any cell in the body. Essentially, when they get a signal, usually from a kind of hormone, they grow or mature into their end form. There are two basic types of stem cells: embryonic and adult forms.

Embryonic stem cells are usually obtained with permission from fertility clinics when a fertilised egg has divided a few times to form a little ball of stem cells called a zygote. These cells are truly blank canvases and can make virtually any cell in the body. However, they're difficult to come across and, as you can imagine, they are subjected to tight regulation and ethical considerations.

Adult stem cells exist in all of us. Probably the best-known type are those that are located in our bone marrow, but in actual fact, we have little stem cells everywhere. For the most part, aside from frequently growing and changing tissues, such as our bone marrow and our gut, stem cells just live there, dormant, for our whole lives.

One exciting development in stem cell research is that scientists have worked out a way to take our own cells backwards in evolution and then regrow them. They are called induced pluripotent stem cells, which essentially translates to stem cells that scientists induce to become nearly anything (pluripotent is 'multiple potentials'). The cells are grown by taking a few millimetres of skin: meaning they are the patient's own – genetically identical.

These ex-skin cells, now stem cells, can be encouraged to turn into cardiac myocytes, or heart muscle cells, genetically identical to the cells that already exist in that person's body. From here, they can be used to fix hearts that are sick. Or at least, they will be able to in the very near future.

Research into stem cells has been a slow growth area until recently when induced stem cells were discovered. The outcomes for research into the use of stem cells for heart disease has been variable. That's not necessarily because stem cells don't work, but because there are so many factors at play that pose a challenge, including growing the cells and delivering them to their destination, and the cells then 'taking' successfully and growing correctly, and finally working correctly.

One of the major challenges is getting the implanted stem cells to survive and grow into the heart correctly. Published in one of the major heart research journals called *Circulation,* a study by a group of heart researchers from Israel found that stem cells living in our heart muscle could cause more inflammation and difficulties with the heart's pumping mechanism when they were induced to act by heart damage itself.

The research is ongoing but it does seem to indicate that eventually we will be able to repair broken hearts by giving them new, healthy cells. The results we have seen so far are promising, and perhaps in the not-too-distant future we will be able to borrow some of the zebra fish magic and regrow and regenerate damaged hearts.

Growing a whole new heart

In the 1990s a photo of a lab mouse that had grown what looked like a human ear on its back circulated around the world, polarising opinions. People were either repulsed or ecstatic. Even though the sight of a mouse carrying around an ear was a little disturbing, I thought it was also undeniably pretty cool. It meant the possibility now existed for science to grow you a replacement finger or ear if you needed one, made from your own cells, that could be sewn on to you. An ear is one thing, possibly a life-changing event, but a new organ could be life-saving. Every year, people die while on the transplant waiting list. A life-saving donor organ does not become available in time for around 22 people per day in the United States. And if you are fortunate enough to receive the precious gift of a new organ, you are committed to a lifetime of drugs that suppress your immune system, hiding it from your body's ever-vigilant immune cells. The body has to be tricked and misled into leaving the new organ alone so that it lives a long and healthy life, along with its recipient.

So what if we could solve two problems at once? Rather than waiting for a donor organ, what if we could grow one? And even better, if we could do it from your own cells so that the heart was literally made of you, we wouldn't have to hide it from your immune system.

Science fiction perhaps? But maybe not for too much longer. In 2017 an American in a Massachusetts lab grew heart cells on a spinach leaf. Which seems odd, I agree. The method is like a recipe so we need to go through it step by step. I promise, the leaf will be important.

Like any good recipe, we need to start with ingredients. This is where the stem cells come in. First of all, we make (or collect) stem cells that can be taught to grow and divide into the cells of the heart, the cardiac myocytes. They can grow and grow but they need to do so in an orderly fashion. They need a scaffold, and that's where the leaf comes in.

Hold a leaf up to the light and you will see a fine network of vessels through it, not dissimilar to what we have in our own bodies. When the heart muscle cells were placed on the leaf, they grew along this natural scaffold. They were guided and well constrained by this kind of trellis that the leaf had given them. In other biological settings where organs or tissues are grown, the scaffold can be many other things, including plastic.

The leaf also served another important function, which was to behave like the blood vessels of the heart. Blood vessels inside the heart are incredibly fine and can be very difficult to replicate in a lab setting. The heart depends on blood vessels as small as 10 microns (a tenth of a millimetre) to keep it alive. The humble spinach leaf may have helped solve one of modern research's biggest dilemmas.

For me, one of the most fascinating aspects of the heart is the way heart muscle cells just beat. As simple as that. By themselves, in a group or in a heart, when heart muscle cells are given life-sustaining nutrients such as oxygen, glucose and fatty acids, they do exactly what nature intended: they contract rhythmically.

It's quite a stretch to go from creating heart cells that live and beat together on a leaf or some other scaffold to making a whole heart. For one thing, the heart is not just made of muscle but dozens of other kinds of cells, including those that make the blood vessels, valves and the electrical system of the heart. Not only do we need to make and grow those cells but we need to get those cells to all mix together in the correct numbers and then grow together in an orderly fashion to create a heart.

Now it seems as though we are really getting into science-fiction land. In reality, it may not be too far away. The fact that researchers can grow heart cells that can beat together functionally is a huge hurdle that has already been overcome. At the very least we are close to being able to grow parts of hearts, such as muscle or heart valves to replace damaged sections. In labs and hospitals around the world, the ability to fix a broken heart may not be as far away as we think.

What would this mean? Well for one, being able to replace whole sections of a damaged heart could restore normal function to the heart as a whole. That would translate to not just restoring the heart but perhaps someone's life. If a heart transplant was needed, it could come from a lab rather than another person who has died. It might mean the end of suppressing immune systems because the heart would be made just for you.

'Vaccine' against heart disease

Treating cholesterol can be difficult. As many of us know from personal experience, using diet to lose weight or lower cholesterol can be hard for many reasons. We have medication that is effective in lowering cholesterol but it can come with side effects that make it difficult to take for long periods of time. Plus, not everyone is great at taking medicines every day.

Early in 2017 a group from Harvard and the University of Pennsylvania published some exciting work that was hailed as a kind of vaccine against heart disease. Essentially they worked out a way to give rats a single injection that reduced levels of LDL (bad) cholesterol for good.

A gene called 'PCSK9' was discovered in families that have high rates of heart attack and it seemed to be responsible for regulating bad cholesterol. This gene can prevent cholesterol being removed from the bloodstream and packed away somewhere safe where it can't injure blood vessels or hearts. This 'vaccine' targeted this gene to stop it from keeping cholesterol in the bloodstream. While not technically a vaccine, it acted like one, with one injection offering huge protection. In mice, the levels of cholesterol dropped by enough to translate to reducing the risk of heart attack by up to 90 per cent in humans. A new drug like this has some testing and research ahead of it to ensure it's both safe and effective for humans. Despite that, it's an exciting development.

New medications are being researched and developed all the time. We are also learning that different medications affect different people in a multitude of ways. For some, medications are incredibly effective and life-saving. For others, they don't work as well and have side effects. Aspirin is a great example of a drug that has been life-saving for many hearts but not for others; some people still have heart attacks while taking aspirin.

The future is bright when it comes to creating super-specialised and highly effective drugs. It may revolve around individualised medicine, whereby through genetic testing or some other lab-based testing, we doctors can prescribe exactly the right drugs for the person sitting in front of us.

The diabetes and obesity epidemic

When I was a kid, I remember hearing about starving children around the world. Our TV screens were filled with pictures of small children from lands far away, with pot bellies, starving in some of the poorest communities. In African countries, diseases such as diabetes and obesity were virtually unheard of. Unlike the people in most Western countries who were feeding themselves into early graves, those in the poorest countries of the world could not afford to buy or make enough food to sustain themselves.

While people around the world still suffer from starvation and malnutrition, there is change afoot. Now, disease due to an excess of food is more common than disease due to an inadequate food supply. Diseases that were primarily found in the West are now being seen in some of the world's poorest countries in Africa, South

America and Asia. The World Health Organisation has listed obesity as one of the most pressing public health issues of our time.

In 1980 the WHO reported that the number of people worldwide with diabetes was 108 million. Now there are at least 422 million people worldwide with diabetes. These people are two or three times more likely to have strokes or heart attacks. In the same timeframe, the number of overweight and obese adults has more than doubled around the world. More people now live in countries where being overweight is a problem than live in countries where malnutrition is the most pressing issue.

It's not as though we're staying on an even keel in the prosperous West. When I was a medical student, we learnt about diabetes. There was type 1 diabetes, almost universally a disease of childhood and adolescence where the pancreas was damaged and didn't make enough insulin. Type 2 diabetes, on the other hand, occurred mainly due to lifestyle – inactivity and poor diet – whereby the body made enough insulin but the tissues couldn't respond and grab excess sugar from the bloodstream. Type 2 diabetes was largely a disease of older, overweight adults.

Since I left medical school, this has changed. Now a child with diabetes may have the 'adult' form of type 2 diabetes, in which their body acts like that of an adult who has subjected their body to years of a poor lifestyle. At the same time, the overall global burden created by diabetes, obesity and high blood pressure continues to rise. This can only mean bad news for the heart.

If we don't address this rapidly rising rate of diabetes and obesity, an impending explosion of heart disease and its close cousin, stroke, is coming our way. If there is a good, a bad and an ugly to the future of our hearts, this is absolutely the ugly. Many suggestions have been proposed to engage each and every one of us in looking after ourselves by making better food choices and being more physically active.

Healthy societies

When a health issue is of great importance to our whole society – in every sense, from wellbeing to economic – we enlist public health measures to tackle a problem. The two best examples of these kinds of public health measures were campaigns tackling vaccination and smoking. Vaccination was introduced to many, many people to eradicate and control diseases such as polio and smallpox (among dozens of others) that created an enormous strain on our healthcare system and killed or injured vast numbers of people worldwide.

Smoking control was another very successful public health campaign. If this book had been written in the 1950s or 1960s, I may have included a piece on my favourite kind of cigarette, including which ones were healthier for you! Thankfully we've moved on and rather than endorsing tobacco, doctors fight vigorously against it. Decreasing smoking rates had a great impact on the rates of heart disease and a number of types of cancer, such as lung cancer.

With growing epidemics of obesity and diabetes threatening the health and wellbeing of hearts around the globe, public health measures are constantly up for discussion. From positive measures such as creating parks and sports facilities or not taxing fresh fruit and vegetables, to deterrents such as taxing sugar, tobacco and even car usage, governments at every level in every country will need to start throwing everything they have at this tidal wave of disease. Stem cells and spinach leaves may be our future, but prevention is far and away the best medicine.

A doctor on your wrist

Confession: I am a gadget junkie. I can't help it: I get sucked in by the marketing and then all of a sudden I find myself unable to live without my latest gadget. I may be able to justify my latest obsession though, as it could tell me whether my heart is healthy or not.

The Apple Watch was released to much fanfare, as are a lot of Apple products. One of the major selling points was that it had built-in health applications, including tracking your sleep and encouraging you to exercise. In fact, the Apple Watch is one of many wearable devices on the market that is geared towards keeping you healthy, with reminders and trackers to show and celebrate your achievements.

An app specifically designed for the Apple Watch can receive data all day about its owner's heart rate and rhythm. The common heart rhythm problem called atrial fibrillation, which as we've discussed can often be asymptomatic but have important consequences for the heart, is one problem the device hopes to address. Atrial fibrillation cuts off blood supply and can lead to stroke. The app recognises this and in the future will be able to alert a user that they need to see a doctor.

This is a pretty basic level of detection; however, it was something that we previously didn't have the ability to detect or screen for in this way. In the future, with more apps and more wearable technology available to us all, we may be able to detect heart disease earlier, treat it earlier and prevent its progression to more serious disease.

The ability to reliably monitor our hearts in our own homes or on our wrists and then report back to medical professionals is something we can do now. Home monitoring of hearts for people who already have a disease has been a feature of medical devices such as pacemakers for several years. However, home monitoring as a preventative measure is something new. A pacemaker is a kind of battery inserted, usually under the collarbone, with electrical leads that go into the heart, delivering electricity to ensure that it beats at a safe rate. The first pacemaker was made in the same hospitals that pioneered heart surgery. At that time, to move a patient from the operating theatre to a ward bed meant someone had to run from power point to power point down the hall, literally plugging the patient in at every step. Now pacemakers are tiny, with batteries that last up to 10 years. Not only are they 'wireless' but we also have the ability to monitor the pacemaker and the heartbeat and heart rhythm from a transducer at home, which sends the information to the patient's hospital.

It may seem like a natural evolution to have our whole lives on our wrists or in our pockets, and just an extension of the incredible technology we now have available to us. However, as they say, knowledge is power and that is especially true when it comes to heart health. The ability to detect problems early, sometimes even before a patient notices anything wrong, is amazingly powerful. Nobody wants to develop a physical manifestation of their illness too late, and Apple Watches and the endless stream of commercial and medical devices that serve as early warning signs may save lives and enhance our heart health.

Medicine in the age of Dr Google

Science's uncertainty is not its shortcoming, but its strength. Rather than a deficiency of knowledge, not knowing everything is a good way to start knowing more. Even the most elegantly executed research studies raise more questions, and so the process repeats itself. I love that we never stop asking questions and that we never stop learning. There is so much more to discover and with every experiment, every new question, we get better and better answers. Don't be afraid about uncertainty; be excited about what we might learn next! For me, the ability to take all this new and important information and use it in my day job has been such a wonderful way to thank the incredible people who do the research hard yards.

When I started studying medicine, there was so much information that it seemed crazy to imagine there could still be more to discover. Yet since that time, some astounding discoveries have been made and continue to be made. Science is wonderful and ever evolving. Each time we learn something new it creates change that can profoundly improve our lives. It's a very exciting time as we learn more and more about our bodies, about disease and about the wider world.

Knowledge is power but, more importantly, knowing how to interpret or evaluate that knowledge is even more powerful. Understanding that science is a process, and understanding how you can assess that process, is a wonderful tool when you are sifting through vast amounts of health advice. When you can understand what is being said, and why it changes, then you can integrate the important parts into your life for a healthier heart and a happier you.

The internet has given many people a platform to have their voice heard. It's revolutionised the way we learn and teach, and meant that people with something to say don't need expert degrees or public personas to do so. With an internet connection, you have near-instantaneous information exchange. While there isn't anything wrong with spreading the word online without a degree or some other specialisation, it's also easy to receive erroneous information from people who aren't across all of the issues. You don't have to look far to find examples of social media popularising sometimes harmful practices.

Information is everywhere today, easily accessible even from our phones. This avalanche of information brings knowledge to us easily, but it also means that we get a lot of bad with the good. So is this a post doing the rounds on social media, or is it from a reputable news website? Social media does lend itself to limited disclosure of information. When you come across online health advice, it is advisable to ask: who is the person telling me this? Look for their qualifications, their genuine personal experience and any institutions they're affiliated with. If they're writing on behalf of an organisation, dig deeper to find out what that organisation is. Most online sites have an 'About me' section.

Healthcare workers spend many years learning how to properly read and interpret research, picking apart everything to decide whether or not it's worthwhile. There are many secrets hidden away in the often confusing text of a research article. As a reader of that article, whether you're a doctor or the person who might be on the receiving end of that treatment, it's important to unearth all of that information.

Reputable news sources may be more likely to link to the original study. This is incredibly important because to fully assess how good the information is, you need to be able to see the source article. Big health websites such as Harvard Health, WebMD or some government health websites will generally link to the information so that you can properly assess it.

Get curious, read and embrace the change and the science. Question the information and look to reputable sources for advice. I am convinced that if you learn about how wonderful your heart actually is, you will want to love it even more.

Prevention is always better than cure

Prevention is an exciting area in research about our hearts. While fixing broken hearts is vital, stopping them from getting that way is many times better than the best mechanical heart or the most effective medicine. Medicine and surgery of the heart is astonishing, but not nearly as amazing as your own, perfectly healthy heart.

One of the most heartbreaking parts of my jobs is when I see someone whose heart or whole body is too unwell to be fixed. It is exceedingly difficult to have to say, 'I'm sorry, but there isn't any way that we can help you'. Sometimes, a patient is too sick and wouldn't survive an operation. Sometimes, because their disease has become so severe, an operation is not technically possible anymore. In other patients, organ systems like the kidneys have suffered so much damage from the heart disease (or other disease) that an operation would be far too stressful on their body and their chance of making a meaningful recovery with a good quality of life is minimal. It's one of the worst conversations I have to have.

The saying 'an apple a day keeps the doctor away' extols the virtues of prevention. With all of the exciting developments in medicine for the heart, it's hard to keep that in mind. Does that mean that all of these great advances in heart disease treatment are a waste? Should we just forget them and make everyone exercise and eat well? Well, no. Because even with a good lifestyle, good genes or a combination of risks and relievers, some people with still have heart disease. People will continue to smoke, be overweight or develop diabetes for the foreseeable future.

I remember my days at medical school when the fight against disease was often geared around treating it, not preventing it. I wonder if it was a function of the fact that we had so much to get through in a set timeframe or whether the elements of prevention are vastly more complicated than just saying 'eat well'. The science of prevention, including nutrition and exercise, has come a long way. Doctors are taught to fight disease – the very reason that we exist – but prevention doesn't get as much attention as it should. Sometimes it feels as if we're under a mountain of disease, and it's incredibly hard to find the resources to tackle prevention with any real commitment.

In the United States, healthcare spending on prevention accounts for less than 5 per cent of money thrown at health. That is a tiny amount. Yet some estimates show that if we reduce our energy (food) consumption by just 100 kilocalories a day, we can potentially reduce the cases of obesity by 71 million people. That's almost triple the population of Australia. The maths is not perfect and involves a lot of extrapolation, but nonetheless, even relatively small changes can have major effects around the world.

Prevention makes good sense and it makes good cents. The responsibility for prevention falls to all of us, from governments and the private sector to us as individuals. The thing is this: diseases can be untreatable. They can be more easily treated when they're discovered earlier. Disease can also be prevented, and this should be our long game.

I'm excited for the future of medicine, by the prospect of new operations or different and better tests. The idea of looking at your wrist and knowing that your heart is healthy is both exciting and reassuring. More than that though, I am excited by prevention. I am excited by the possibility of a population of empowered people who take good care of themselves, who are determined to prevent this tidal wave of heart disease so that they hopefully never have to meet me in my operating theatre.

Whether it be prevention, stem cells or mechanical hearts, the future of our hearts is bright. Just how bright is hard to predict. Science is always running along in leaps and bounds and public policy needs to join it. Perhaps in another 10 years we will be talking about issues that are barely even an idea in some clever person's mind right now. Investing in our own hearts and investing in the research for all of our hearts is, without a doubt, one of the best outlays we will ever make.

INDEX